seductive delusions

seductive*

delusions

How Everyday People Catch STDs

JILL GRIMES, M.D.

The Johns Hopkins University Press
Baltimore

Note to the Reader: This book presents accounts of people who have a sexually transmitted disease. None of the characters portrayed here are actual people; any resemblance to actual people is purely coincidental.

This book also covers symptoms, diagnosis, and treatment for readers who are concerned that they may be infected or who are infected. It is not meant to substitute for medical care of people with an STD, and treatment should not be based solely on its contents. Treatment must be developed in a dialogue between the individual and his or her physician. This book has been written to help with that dialogue.

Drug dosage: The author and publisher have made reasonable efforts to determine that the selection and dosage of drugs discussed in this text conform to the practices of the medical community. The medications described do not necessarily have specific approval by the U.S. Food and Drug Administration for use in the diseases and dosages for which they are recommended. In view of ongoing research, changes in government regulations, and the constant flow of information relating to drug therapy and drug reactions, the reader is urged to check the package insert of each drug for any change in indications and dosage and for warnings and precautions, particularly when the recommended agent is a new and/ or infrequently used drug.

© 2008 The Johns Hopkins University Press
All rights reserved. Published 2008
Printed in the United States of America on acid-free paper
9 8 7 6 5 4 3 2 1

The Johns Hopkins University Press
2715 North Charles Street
Baltimore, Maryland 21218-4363
www.press.jhu.edu

Library of Congress Cataloguing-in-Publication Data will be found at the end of this book.

A catalog record for this book is available from the British Library.

ISBN-13: 978-0-8018-9066-6 (hc)
ISBN-13: 978-0-8018-9067-3 (pbk)
ISBN-10: 0-8018-9066-7 (hc)
ISBN-10: 0-8018-9067-5 (pbk)

Special discounts are available for bulk purchases of this book. For more information, please contact Special Sales at 410-516-6936 or specialsales@press.jhu.edu.

The Johns Hopkins University Press uses environmentally friendly book materials, including recycled text paper that is composed of at least 30 percent post-consumer waste, whenever possible. All of our book papers are acid-free, and our jackets and covers are printed on paper with recycled content.

To all my patients,
in thanks for your trust

Contents

Preface

I LOVE BEING A FAMILY physician, because it is such a thoroughly challenging and rewarding career. People come in hurting or ill, and they trust me to help them. Sometimes it's simple—a strep throat that is easily fixed with an antibiotic. Often, it's more complex, involving multiple diseases such as diabetes and heart disease. While medications help to control and treat these problems, lifestyle changes have an enormous influence on health. It is very gratifying for doctors to teach our patients proper diet and exercise. This education empowers our patients to fix the baseline problem, for example, obesity, rather than simply treating its complications. Of course, in primary care, our goal is always to give our patients such tools before they develop a disease, to *prevent* rather than *treat* disease and illness.

One frustration that I share with many of my colleagues is our seeming lack of ability to help our patients avoid contracting sexually transmitted diseases. Whether the problem is time constraints or simply less-than-effective communication, we often fall short in this arena. Our patients who are diagnosed with a sexually transmitted disease inevitably look at us in shock and dismay, sincerely wondering how this could possibly have happened to them. Somehow we doctors, as well as textbooks and classroom lessons teaching basic principles for preventing the spread of STDs, are failing. Universally, there is a seductive delusion that if we choose the "right" people, there won't be any adverse emotional or physical consequences from sexual activity. No one seems to believe that these fundamental principles *apply to them* or their group of friends.

The media certainly portray STDs as an issue for the social outcasts of our society. Although we hear about new "hookups" between superstars every week, when was the last time we heard of an actor or supermodel catching an STD? No, the common belief is that STDs belong with prostitutes and drug addicts, and not with "people like us." While people who have sex with multiple partners do have higher risks, the population most primary care physicians treat for STDs is not who you might expect. What I want to tell you is that *we discover STDs in everyone* from cheerleaders, valedictorians, and athletes to professionals of all disciplines. No social class, gender, or race is immune.

How can we help people become aware of the risks associated with their sexual activity, when they often believe, erroneously, that they are not at risk? Since sex education and physicians' pamphlets don't seem to get this idea across, I thought I would try a different approach. Stories are far more powerful than statistics. I decided to tell the stories of people I know, patients I see, who are just like you and me—and who get an STD.

If you miss an episode of your favorite television series, your best friend can update you with accurate details of what happened, describing complex relationships and even medical procedures on shows like *Grey's Anatomy* or *ER*. How can they absorb and subsequently relate all that information? They remember all the specifics because they lived through them with the characters—seeing, feeling, and experiencing the action. The details of the show are now a firm memory for them. My hope is that sharing stories of successful, intelligent, attractive women and men as they are stunned with the diagnosis of a sexually transmitted disease will help the reader remember the details of STD prevention as easily as they remember the details of a television series. This information will help them understand that they are at risk and will ultimately help them avoid acquiring an STD, a disease they may have for the rest of their life.

As you begin this book, please keep in mind that you can read all of these stories at one time, or you can start with the STD you are concerned about, whether you are worried that you might already have this STD or that you may get it or give it to someone else. (If you do have such concerns, the best thing you can do is see your physician for testing and advice before you engage in any additional sexual activity.) The story of each disease is told through the perspective of a male and a female character, to allow the reader to identify with his or her own gender (or to gain some understanding of and empathy with what a partner might be experiencing). After each pair of stories, a fact section provides a quick reference for the symptoms, treatment, prevention, and other important information about that STD, as well as answers to frequently asked questions. A list of websites points to additional information.

Your sexual health today has implications that range far into the future. Decisions made early in your life regarding sexual activity can impact future fertility, self-worth, and even choice of a life partner. No one sets out thinking they are going to catch any disease, but *you can't go back and make a different decision* once you've contracted a viral STD or developed scarring in your reproductive organs.

In an attempt to respect our patients' choices, we doctors may not do enough to describe the potential emotional hazards of sexual encounters. The decision to be sexually intimate should involve much more than the knowledge of how to prevent pregnancy and how to avoid STDs.

Healthy relationships thrive on open communication, mutual respect, and trust. These qualities should apply universally, including to discussions and decisions about physical intimacy. Understanding the emotional and physical consequences of sexual activity helps empower people to talk meaningfully and honestly with a prospective partner before impulsively reacting to hormones, perceived expectations, passion, or even true love.

I wrote this book because I worry about every patient who has agonized in my office when I told them that they have a sexually transmitted disease. Unfortunately, I have seen hundreds of patients with STDs for every one patient portrayed in this book. (As such, any resemblance of a character in the book to any specific patient is purely coincidental.) Many of the medical issues described here can apply to STDs acquired through homosexual as well as heterosexual intimacy. I have not included stories about gay men or lesbians, however, because I did not find a reasonable way to make the book representative without making it twice as long. Information for homosexual partners is included in the facts and frequently asked questions sections of the book.

Pregnancy is not addressed in this book, although it is clearly another potential consequence of unplanned or unprotected sex. While an unplanned pregnancy can bring joy (sometimes unexpected joy), it also can cause anguish. This book, as the title states, focuses on how people catch sexually transmitted diseases.

After reading the fact sections after each disease, readers may question the effectiveness of condoms in preventing disease. Condoms have been proven to work best for decreasing transmission of STDs carried through semen—HIV, chlamydia, gonorrhea, and trichomonas. They do not offer the same level of protection against diseases transmitted through direct contact such as herpes, HPV, syphilis, and pubic lice. To be maximally effective, condoms must be used consistently, correctly, and for all types of genital contact, including oral-genital. Breakage, slippage, inconsistent and improper use (such as putting on after pre-ejaculate has occurred) lead to condom failure rates of nearly twenty percent.

I learned long ago not to judge people, and I hope this book reflects my intent to create a non-moralistic approach to the problem of STDs. This is not a book that says you're bad if you have sex. It is a practical, informative book that says look, here are the facts about what you risk medically if you have sex. I hope that you learn and benefit from the experiences depicted in this book and use them to protect yourself, your friends, and your loved ones.

Many wonderful people deserve thanks. First is my dear friend, Frank Domino, M.D., for his enthusiastic support from the very first story, before there was a book, to confirming medical accuracy at the end. Next is lifelong friend Stephanie Carinci, M.D., who encouraged me to grab even ten-minute scraps of time to write every day. Brilliant fiction author and friend Jeff Abbott provided so much help, from his basic advice to all aspiring authors, "write the book," to nitty-gritty details of font and type size, giving me all the tools I needed to get off the ground. To Jeff and his wife, Leslie, thanks for your invaluable support. To author and doctor Ari Brown, M.D., thanks for your interest and guidance along this exciting path.

Lynn, Rich, and Elise read very early versions, and prompted me to continue work when I stalled. Other friends listened to my ideas and gave me valuable feedback, laughs, and zeal to continue— special thanks to Coni, Terri, Lorna, Barbara, Suzanne, Catherine, and Mary. To my Crested Butte buddies, Christel and Dr. Joanne, I appreciate your joy and celebration of the book contract. Fellow "mommydocs" cheered every step of the way, especially Dr. Ann, Dr. Julia, and Dr. Susan.

I thank all my wonderful patients for trusting me with the care of their health, especially those families I have had the privilege of knowing and treating for many years. I appreciate the support of all the doctors and staff at West Lake Family Practice. Drs. Eunice Chen, Kristyn Fagerberg, Scott Gaertner, and Cary Douglass make the practice of medicine the way it should be—rewarding, challenging, and fun.

I now understand why authors thank their editors. Huge thanks to Jacqueline Wehmueller for always staying positive, listening to my concerns, and expertly streamlining stories. Copy editor Susan Lantz had an amazing eye for sorting details of confusing medical statistics and flow of dialogue. I'm grateful to you both.

To Mom in heaven and Dad, "ye ole professor" here on earth, thanks for my love of books and desire to teach. To Bene, my sweet R.N. mother-in-law, much love. To my sister, Linda, thanks for sharing your expertise as a gynecologist. To John and the rest of our family, love and thanks. To our wonderful daughters, Brittany and

Nicole, thanks for cheering me on when you're not even old enough to understand the content of this book. Finally, to my incredible husband, Drew, who prioritized my writing at the sacrifice of his needs and who believes in me one hundred percent—I love you.

seductive delusions

HERPES SIMPLEX VIRUS

1: Elaine

"THE DOCTOR WILL BE in to see you shortly," said the perky medical assistant at the university health center. That was nearly twenty minutes ago. Long enough for Elaine to flip through all of the dated *People* magazines, memorize the stop smoking poster, and count the tiles in the floor. It was also long enough for the sweat on the back of her thighs to soak the paper on the exam table, causing it to stick to her and rip as she shifted nervously. Elaine fretfully twirled a strand of her straight, shoulder-length blond hair. She was freezing in this paper-thin gown, yet anxiety was making her perspire. How could she have ended up in this spot? As a medical student, she was already feeling as though she belonged on the other side of the exam table.

Her thoughts drifted back to that first day in class. The professor was finishing up his introduction to the trials and tribulations of medical school, and he had one final admonition. "Remember, do not date your classmates. You will be working side by side with these people for the next four years—sleep deprived, mentally and physically exhausted. Believe me, you don't need the extra emotional baggage that these relationships will bring." Everyone shared a good laugh. But by the end of the first month, almost half of the class was romantically involved, and Elaine was no exception.

In the gross anatomy lab, four students were assigned to each cadaver. Elaine was paired up with James on the right side of the body, and two other classmates had the left side. James's sense of humor attracted Elaine, although he was not her usual physical type. Both of Elaine's former college boyfriends had been very tall, thin, and wiry. In contrast, James was only around five foot nine, which was about three inches taller than Elaine, with an extremely muscular build that reflected his frequent competition in triathlons. Elaine and James had immediate chemistry. Their rush of nervous adrenaline from that first day of actually dissecting a human body had carried them into a quickly deepening relationship—first study partners, then partners in bed. Elaine had been shocked by how fast they had ended up sleeping together. She was not a virgin, but had only had sex with two other men in her life, both long-term college boyfriends. It must have been the high of everything coming together in her life. She had always dreamed of becoming a doctor, and now here she was in her first year of medical school. She was bursting with confidence and excitement. James shared these same passions, and an enthusiastic hug and kiss at the end of their first round of practice exams had turned passionate. Now they had been together almost six months.

Last month, just after her period, Elaine had developed an incredibly painful sore in her crotch. She had been certain that it was a pressure sore from her new jeans. Elaine bought them because she loved the flowers stitched down the sides, but she had hoped they would stretch out a bit, since they were a little too snug. As she sat through the long eight-hour days of lectures, followed by many more hours in the library or at James's condo studying for their exams, a seam in the jeans must have rubbed a sore spot. However, when the sore area began to ache and burn again after her period this month, Elaine was afraid this sore had nothing to do with her jeans. So here she sat at her gynecologist's office, dreading the upcoming exam.

A rattle at the door as the doctor grabbed her chart from the door rack told Elaine it was finally her turn.

"Hi. I'm Dr. Chen. So what seems to be the problem today?"

said the doctor as she walked in. Elaine couldn't believe how young her doctor looked. Elaine felt like Dr. Chen should be one of her classmates, rather than her doctor, but overall just was relieved that the doctor was female. Seeing a male doctor for a pelvic exam would have been way too embarrassing.

Elaine took a deep breath to compose herself, wanting to appear cool and intelligent. "Well, I appear to have a recurring painful red sore. I noticed it for the first time last month, right after my period. It lasted around a week or so, and I thought it was from wearing some new jeans. Unfortunately, it came back this month in the same spot, and now I'm worried that it might be . . ."

"Herpes?" filled in Dr. Chen.

Elaine burst into tears. How humiliating. She could barely choke out a reply. "Yes, of course, that's what I'm afraid that it is."

Dr. Chen handed her a tissue and smiled reassuringly. "Let me ask you a few questions, and then we'll take a look."

Elaine sniffed and nodded her head in reply.

"Okay," said Dr. Chen, "have you ever had a sexually transmitted disease before?" A fresh wave of tears washed over Elaine.

"No. I've only had two previous partners, and I have never even had a yeast infection."

Dr. Chen smiled. "Sorry. I know these are very personal questions," she said, "but it's important that I get your past history before I examine you. What kind of birth control are you using?"

"I'm on the pill," Elaine replied.

"Are you using condoms as well?" asked the doctor.

"No, at least, not consistently," Elaine answered, somewhat embarrassed.

"Does your partner have any history of herpes or other sexually transmitted diseases?" said Dr. Chen.

Elaine swallowed. How could she admit that she hadn't had the guts to even tell James about her sore, much less ask him if he had any diseases? Sitting here, it was hard to believe that she would have had sex with someone without knowing everything about his past. She had initially insisted on condoms to "cover" that possibility, but a few times there weren't any handy, and they had sex anyway. "Um, not that I'm aware of."

Dr. Chen looked up at that response but didn't comment. "Okay. Last month, when you first noticed the sore, did you feel sick at all or have any fever?" asked the doctor.

Elaine replied that she had been so busy and tired from studying, she didn't recall being particularly ill, just extremely uncomfortable from the sore.

"Have you put any creams or over-the-counter ointments on the sore?"

"No."

"All right, then. Let's go ahead and take a look."

Elaine took a deep breath as she leaned backward and began to scoot down the exam table. Yet another fresh wave of tears filled her eyes. "Please let me be wrong," she thought. "Please, please, please. I don't want a disease that is going to stay with me the rest of my life. Maybe I'm just being paranoid." After all, "medical student disease" was a common phenomenon in her classmates these days. Whatever disease they studied, several students began to believe that they were suffering from it. Of course, the common symptoms of many diseases, like fatigue, headache, weight gain, or bowel changes, were occurring in every student from the stress of school, but..."

"Okay, let's get your feet in these stirrups," said the doctor, pulling out and positioning the hidden metal supports at the base of the exam table. Dr. Chen's voice snapped Elaine back to reality, and she placed her feet one at a time in the sock-covered stirrups. She felt the heat from the lamp and squeezed her eyes shut. "Just relax," the doctor said.

Elaine almost laughed. She had to remember never to tell a patient that. How could anyone possibly relax at this point?

"Oh." the doctor said. "Is this the spot you were talking about?" Elaine opened her eyes.

"Yes, that's it. What do you think?"

"Well, I'm sorry, but honestly, it does look like herpes. What I'm seeing is a cluster of about five little blisters, which are starting to crust over, and the edge is bright red. I'm going to do a viral culture to confirm it, but I think we should start treatment while we're waiting for the results." Elaine's heart sank. Dr. Chen reached for a metal instrument that Elaine recognized as a speculum and inserted it deftly, saying, "Elaine, I'm going to take a quick look at your cervix and make sure there aren't any additional lesions inside." Elaine tried to focus on the memory of one of her classmates using a speculum as a pretend duck puppet, opening and closing the "bills" of the tool and quacking. Before long, the doctor had removed the instrument and was pressing around the outside portion of Elaine's pelvis.

"You still have some enlarged lymph nodes down here, did you realize that? Feel right here." Elaine obediently reached down and was surprised to feel a tender knot in her right groin. "Okay, you can scoot back and sit up. Let me step out and grab some handouts for you while you get dressed. I'll be right back in to finish talking with you."

Elaine did not feel fully conscious as she went through the motions of getting dressed. Herpes. The "gift that keeps on giving," as one of her classmates so eloquently put it. "Oh my gosh, how am I going to tell James? Actually, he is the one who had better be apologizing to me, since I've never had an outbreak before. What a jerk. I am going to strangle him when I . . ."

A quick knock interrupted her thoughts. "Are you dressed?" asked Dr. Chen.

"Yes, come in," replied Elaine.

"Okay, I'm going to talk to you as though you were not a medical student, and just give you my standard speech so I'm sure that I told you everything, without assuming that you know all about this, okay?"

Elaine felt on the verge of tears again, so she simply nodded in agreement.

"All right, your sores do look like herpes. In a couple of days, we'll get results from the tests that I took, and then we'll know for certain." Dr. Chen stopped a moment to hand Elaine a tissue, and then she continued. "Many people want to know if it is 'type one' or 'type two,' but I did not order that test because it will not change how we treat you. It used to be that type one herpes was oral, and type two was genital. We believe that somewhere between fifty and eighty percent of people living in the United States have been infected with oral herpes by the age of twenty, whether they actively break out with sores or not."

"Do you mean sexually active adults, or all adults?" Elaine asked.

"All adults. Much of herpes simplex type one, which we abbreviate as HSV type one, is transmitted in childhood by kissing or sharing cups or utensils with infected adults in the home. Anyway, given the frequency of oral herpes, it shouldn't surprise you to learn that now we see an increase in the number of cases of genital herpes that are actually type one, transmitted through oral sex. Studies show that newly diagnosed genital herpes is HSV type one in anywhere from thirty to seventy percent of the cases. Some people abstain from genital sex in the hopes of avoiding sexually transmittable diseases and then, ironically, they end up here with genital herpes as the result of one partner passing on herpes from their mouth to the other partner's genitals. Also, while many people use condoms with genital intercourse, fewer people use them with oral sex."

Elaine nodded to show she was listening, but inside, her head was swimming with questions. Did James know he had herpes? Why didn't she insist on condoms? Why didn't he? How could they have been so careless?

The doctor continued, "Anyway, we do have antiviral drugs that really help a great deal with herpes. Unfortunately, we don't have anything yet that completely eradicates the disease, but at least they can make outbreaks go away more quickly. We're going to get you started on one today, in fact. There are several different brands, but in general, they work roughly the same. I brought you some samples of valacyclovir—Valtrex is its brand name. You'll take one pill twice per day for three days. The medicine is usually well tolerated, but some people experience some stomach upset or headache. I'm also going to give you a prescription. To begin with, you'll just take the medicine whenever you have an outbreak. It's important to start the medicine as soon as you notice anything. Many people have a sensation of burning, tingling, or itching before they actually break out with the blisters. If you do get that, be sure to start taking the medicine at the first hint of your symptoms. The sooner into the outbreak that you start taking the medicine, the shorter the duration of the outbreak."

Elaine interrupted, "So if I start the medicine right away, how long do you think I'll have these blisters?"

"Typically, they last around four or five days, but everyone is different," the doctor replied.

"How frequently do you think I'll break out?" Elaine asked, her voice tremulous.

Dr. Chen frowned. "I wish I could tell you infrequently, but I have to say that with the mental and physical stress of med school, I would bet that you may have frequent outbreaks the first year or two. You've already established an early pattern of breaking out around your period, right?"

"Well, in retrospect, yes. But this is only my second outbreak."

"Well, if it turns out that you are having frequent outbreaks, I think we should put you on suppressive therapy, instead of just treating eruptions."

"What does that mean?" asked Elaine.

"We put you on a once-a-day dose as prevention, in the hopes that it will keep the virus dormant and you won't have outbreaks," said Dr. Chen.

"Why don't we just do that from the beginning, then?" asked Elaine.

"Well, actually, I guess we could. To be honest, the main reason I wouldn't suggest it right now is that the cost is not cheap. If you were like I was in medical school, it would be tough to justify the expense of daily therapy until you see a true pattern of how often you're going to break out," she answered.

"How much money are we talking about?" asked Elaine.

"It depends on your insurance, so I can't tell you exactly, but without any insurance, the newer anti-herpes drugs that you only have to take twice a day for three to five days can cost around sixty dollars per treatment. If you were taking it daily for suppressive treatment, that would be about two hundred dollars per month."

"Oh my gosh—I totally cannot afford that," gasped Elaine. "But I think I just have a co-pay with my prescriptions. I think it's like fifteen dollars if it's generic, and thirty-five if it's name brand."

"You're lucky—with my insurance, the co-pay for prescriptions starts at thirty bucks for the generic. Anyway, it depends what's on the formulary for your insurance. Every insurance company has their own contracts with the drug companies, so whether you only have to pay your co-pay just depends on which ones are on the preferred list for your company. I already wrote you a script for the famciclovir, like the samples I gave you, but I'll also write one for acyclovir, or Zovirax. It's older and less expensive, and you take it three times per day. You can decide which one you want to take based on what your insurance company says," said Dr. Chen.

"Can you give me samples of both so I can see if there's any difference in side effects?" asked Elaine.

"No, I'm sorry. Since acyclovir is now generic, we don't get samples any more. The drug companies just tend to leave samples of the newest medicines," she replied.

"Oh, I understand. Thanks for these samples, I really appreciate it," Elaine responded.

Dr. Chen continued her discourse on the variable manifestations of herpes. "Anyway, you should know that some people are so sensitive that they cannot even wear jeans for a year or so because anything rubbing in the area causes an outbreak. Other people have one or two outbreaks then don't have another for a very long time. The herpes virus likes to pick one nerve pathway to come out on, so people tend break out in the same spot, or at least on the same side in roughly the same spot, each time."

Dr. Chen grimaced slightly as she went on, "In my clinical experience, women have the worse end of the deal. Periods are a very common trigger for outbreaks, so obviously that alone makes it worse for females. People under a lot of stress of any kind—nutritional, sleep, physical, or mental stress—tend to have more frequent outbreaks. We'll just have to see how you do, and how you tolerate the medicine, before we can make an intelligent decision about how to treat you. Does that make sense?"

"Yes, I guess so," agreed Elaine.

Dr. Chen was writing in her chart. Elaine waited until the doctor appeared to be finished with her writing and then asked the question that had been bothering her most: "Is there anything else I need to know about herpes? I mean, can this affect me down the road when I want to have kids?"

Dr. Chen put down her pen. "Well," she replied, "it really shouldn't affect your ability to conceive. Other STDs like chlamydia and gonorrhea can certainly cause scarring of the fallopian tubes and lead to infertility, but we really don't see that with herpes. The main issue with pregnancy and herpes is about delivery. If you have an active lesion when it is time to deliver, we do C-sections instead of vaginal deliveries. Does that answer your question?" Elaine nodded yes.

"And speaking of other STDs, I also did another test on you during the pelvic exam, which checks for chlamydia and gonorrhea. Any time you have one STD, we always check for others. Unfortunately, STDs seem to like to travel in packs, as we say. When you get one, you frequently get another at the same time. So, I should suggest that we draw your blood and screen for HIV. You'll also need to sign a consent form for that, by the way. We should have the results from all your tests in a couple of days. Our nurse will call you when we've got them back. Do you have any other questions about herpes in general?" the doctor asked.

"Yes, one more that I can think of right now. Is there anything, uh, holistic, or whatever, that I can do to make herpes better? You know, like take extra vitamins?" Elaine asked.

"Oh, I'm glad you asked that. If you get on the Internet or look in any health food store, you'll find a million remedies said to prevent herpes outbreaks. The only successful one that I'm aware of from my own clinical experience with my patients over the years is taking lysine daily, which seems to help prevent outbreaks," she said.

"Lysine—that's an amino acid, isn't it? How does that work?" asked Elaine.

Dr. Chen shrugged, "I don't think anyone knows exactly, but I can tell you that I do have some patients that swear by it. They take one hundred milligrams per day to help prevent outbreaks, then triple the dose during any outbreaks."

"Got it," said Elaine. "I guess my only other questions are about transmission. When am I contagious? Just when I can see or feel the blisters?"

"No. Unfortunately, doctors used to think that it was only contagious during outbreaks. Now we know that you can shed virus, and therefore infect someone else, even when you cannot see or feel anything. So, ultimately, you really need to use condoms from now on, because they reduce the risk of transmitting herpes."

"Only reduce the risk?" Elaine questioned.

"Yes, because they cannot cover all the areas where the virus can be transmitted."

"So, I'll need to use condoms forever?"

"Or at least until you're married and trying to conceive."

"And if my future husband doesn't have herpes? What are the chances that I'll pass it on to him if at that point, presumably years from now, if I'm no longer having many or, I hope, any outbreaks?" asked Elaine tentatively.

"Again, I don't have an exact statistic for you. I can tell you that some long-term sexual partners of people with herpes never break out, so it's not one hundred percent, anyway," replied Dr. Chen.

"Well, that's good, but I guess now I'm still obligated to tell anyone that I'm intimate with that I've got herpes, even if I plan to always use condoms."

"Yes," affirmed Dr. Chen. "Unfortunately, many people are either too embarrassed or just plain dishonest, and they pass on all kinds of sexually transmitted diseases because they don't tell their significant others. I know it's hard to share that kind of information, but it's really important."

The doctor stood up and handed Elaine her paperwork so she could check out. "Okay, you should be hearing from us by the end of the week with your test results. Let's hope we won't need to treat anything else, but if we do, we'll bring you back in and take care of it. If you have any more problems, or you start having frequent breakouts, come back in and we'll change you over to daily therapy."

"Okay, thanks," said Elaine. She had actually begun feeling a little better during their conversation, until the doctor mentioned treating anything else. Anything else? As if this weren't bad enough. Tears welled up in her eyes as she gathered up her purse and coat. Herpes. I've got to tell James I've got herpes. No, not I—*we've* got herpes. Oh great, this really was going to be hard. Should she yell at him for giving her herpes? Her heart sunk. It really didn't matter.

Ultimately what mattered to Elaine was that she had genital herpes, now and forever. She'd just have to get past it. "Maybe," she thought sadly, "maybe this will make me a better doctor. A little more compassionate, less judgmental...oh man, this was not exactly how I had expected to learn about sexually transmitted diseases."

2: Justin

SUNDAY MORNING TRAINING RIDES were always the best. Few cars, clear blue skies, birds screeching greetings, and Lake Austin glistening in the early light under the Loop 360 bridge presented an amazing backdrop for the cycling group as they drafted behind one another. Justin's legs burned as he powered up the long, steep hill, sweat pouring down his forehead and stinging his eyes. The adrenaline surge kicked his heart into high gear, racing hard to fuel his screaming legs. Justin imagined himself competing in the Tour de France, pulling for his team like his hero and fellow Austinite, Lance Armstrong. With his fantasy crowds cheering him on, Justin stood up on his pedals, pumping his legs madly for the final hundred meters as his training team crested the hill, all physically exhausted but emotionally charged up with the sheer joy of the ride.

As he reached the top, Justin dropped back onto the saddle of his bike and unexpectedly winced in pain. It was as though a Mack truck had run over him, instantly deflating the joy that had welled up in his chest. "Not again," he agonized.

At five foot eleven, 170 pounds of wiry muscle and virtually no body fat, he looked to be the very picture of health. Justin's lopsided smile, deep blue eyes, and dark brown hair completed the all-American image. In truth, Justin was in excellent physical condition, with one exception. Justin had genital herpes.

His first outbreak of herpes happened in Justin's junior year of high school. Although he had not had "real" sex, Justin developed herpes after receiving oral sex from his girlfriend, Sarah. The first outbreak was the worst, complete with body aches, fever, and amazingly painful blisters covering the right side of the tip of his penis. To add insult to injury, Sarah refused to believe that she had been the source of this pain.

Sarah had always been jealous of the relationship between Justin and his neighbor, Emily. Justin and Emily had grown up together, their friendship dating all the way back to diapers. Justin could never think of Emily as anything beyond a sister, but the intimacy of this lifelong familiarity was threatening to Sarah, who often missed out on inside jokes. Sarah was convinced that Justin had cheated on her with Emily when their two families had gone to the lake together on a weekend Sarah wasn't available. Coincidentally, it was just a few weeks later that Justin developed his first outbreak of herpes. When he told Sarah about it, her immediate reaction was that this sexually transmitted disease offered irrefutable proof of her concerns. Justin was so wounded by her mistrust and false accusations that he didn't bother to fully explain and instead simply broke up with Sarah.

Over the next few years, Justin dated casually, but avoided physical intimacy altogether. Frankly, he wasn't wildly attracted enough to any girl to merit suffering through the embarrassment of explaining that he had herpes. It was far easier to stay superficial, hanging around in groups more than dating exclusively. At least, that had been the case until now.

Justin smiled at Kayla as he walked his bike over to the rack on the back of his Explorer. Her electric-blue-and-purple biking shirt reflected her vibrant personality as it showed off her petite athletic figure. Kayla was twenty, the same age as Justin. Her lightly freckled face was sweaty, and her braided long brown hair was messed up from her helmet, but Justin still thought she looked great.

"That was an awesome ride. I didn't think I was going to make it up that last hill, though," Kayla said, lifting her bike up to the rack behind Justin's.

"No kidding," Justin replied, "my legs feel like rubber. How about yours?"

"Well, let's just say that I'd rather go grab some banana pancakes than go for a run," Kayla laughed.

"Okay, then let's head over to Magnolia Café," suggested Justin. Seeing that Kayla's water bottle had fallen off her bike and rolled to the edge of the parking area, he walked over to grab it for her. As he headed toward the curb, the burning and tingling in his crotch that had started on the ride began to intensify.

Kayla pointed at his legs, saying, "Justin, you weren't kidding about your legs. It looks like you're limping. Are you alright?"

Justin flushed with embarrassment. He realized that he must have been holding his hips off to the side to relieve some of the pressure on his groin. Thank goodness his face was already red and sweaty from the ride, so Kayla didn't notice the difference. For a split second, he thought of actually telling her the truth and just getting it out in the open. Instead, he exaggerated his limp, and in an old man's voice croaked, "Ah, I'm just getting to be too old to ride with cute young things like you. You've crippled me for life." Justin staggered back to the car, and he and Kayla drove off to breakfast.

A few days later, Justin was able to get an appointment to see Dr. Dylan, one of the doctors at the health center on campus.

"So, Justin, what's bothering you today?" asked the doctor.

Justin saw no point in beating around the bush. "Dr. Dylan, as you know, I've had herpes for nearly four years now," he said, pointing to his crotch to indicate which kind of herpes. "I'm really frustrated with these breakouts," he blurted.

"Do you have one now?" he asked.

"Yes, but really that's not my point," Justin said.

"Fair enough. What is your concern?" the doctor countered.

"Well, I'm trying to be healthy. I know that when I'm run down, I break out worse and more often. I'm clear that I need to have regular sleep and eat well, but you know that's not always a choice as a student," Justin said wryly.

"I disagree. I'm not saying it's easy, but it is technically a choice. What's your major?" asked Dr. Dylan.

"Architecture," answered Justin. "When our projects are due, our groups frequently work 'round the clock the last few days."

"Living on pizza and caffeine, no doubt," added Dr. Dylan, with a grin.

"Okay," said Justin defensively, "I get it that finals and project deadlines are going to trigger herpes. I just thought that by now, after four years, it would kind of, well, go away. How much longer do you think I'm going to have to deal with this?"

"Justin, you know we don't have a cure for herpes yet."

"Yes, but usually, doesn't it stop breaking out after awhile?"

"Well, to be honest, in some patients, it does. In others, the out-breaks may continue for decades, and we don't yet know why it affects people so differently," shrugged Dr. Dylan.

"I guess I'm just lucky, then," said Justin sarcastically.

"Well, you're certainly not the worst case I've ever seen, Justin." Dr. Dylan flipped through the chart, looking at previous notes. "You know, I've offered you suppressive therapy before, but you chose not to take it, so I guess it hasn't been that bad, right?"

"It's not that simple. Generally, I feel pretty healthy, and it just seems counterintuitive to take some medicine every day of my life. Do we really know what risks there are from the medicine?" asked Justin.

Dr. Dylan leaned back in his chair. "Well, in all my years of practice, I've never seen any serious complications from the anti-herpes drugs. They are generally very well tolerated. Occasionally people get some nausea or headache, but it's hard to say if that is coming from the drug or actually from the recurrence of herpes. To be honest, I don't know off the top of my head what the manu-facturers of the drug list as the side effects, I just know what I hear complaints about. Here," he grabbed a small book from the counter and flipped through it until he found the medicine he was looking for. "Famvir, famciclovir, lists these short-term complaints as pos-sible side effects: 'Headache—13.5 percent, migraine—0.6 percent, nausea—2.5 percent, diarrhea—4.9 percent, vomiting—1.2 percent, and fatigue—0.6 percent.'"

"And you wonder why I don't want to take it every day?" charged Justin. "What about some of the other medicines that I see ads for? Are they better?"

"In my clinical experience, they all have a similar side-effect pro-file. Also, remember, even placebo is listed at causing headaches, for example, at over five percent. There may be studies that show one drug might be slightly more effective than the others, but mainly it's a matter of patient preference because of how often you have to take the pills or individual side effects. I see your point, but honestly, I rarely have people complain about the medicine causing problems. Usually if they have a complaint, it's about the cost." Dr. Dylan looked expectantly at Justin, "So what do you think? Shall I write you a prescription?" he asked, reaching into his white coat pocket for his prescription pad.

Justin sighed. "Look, I don't mean to be a pain, but I'm not sure. I've got some more questions, if you don't mind."

Dr. Dylan rocked backward again, saying, "Fire away."

"Okay. One thing is, I love to cycle. I've tried a bunch of different sports, but biking is the only thing that I really enjoy and can do consistently. Do you think I'm making the herpes worse with biking?" asked Justin.

"Well, I'd imagine the combination of the tight biking shorts plus the friction against the saddle might aggravate your herpes. It's certainly not the ideal choice for you. Why don't you try running or, better yet, swimming?" Dr. Dylan suggested.

"I tore up my right knee snow skiing last spring break, and it swells up every time I run, so that's out. Swimming is okay, but it's not terribly convenient. It just takes up too much time to head over to the pool or down to the lake to swim."

"Again, it's about choices. What do you think? Have you noticed more breakouts since you started riding?" inquired Dr. Dylan.

"I'm not sure if it causes outbreaks, but if I already have the blisters and I go for any ride longer than thirty or forty minutes, they'll take forever to go away," Justin answered.

"Makes sense, I suppose. Well, why don't you try taking the medicine daily for a few months, and let's see if that will prevent the outbreaks altogether." He again reached for his pad and started to write.

As the doctor wrote out the prescription, Justin realized he had more questions. What he really wanted to ask was when and how in the world should he tell Kayla about his herpes? Dr. Dylan was nice enough, but today he seemed kind of in a hurry. Justin decided on a different tack. "Dr. Dylan, I have a new girlfriend. We haven't, um, done anything yet. I certainly don't want to give her this. If we decide to have sex, what are the chances that she would get herpes from me if I use a condom?"

"Statistics show that if you completely abstain from sex during any outbreaks, and consistently use a condom if you have sex in between breakouts, she will have a ten percent risk of developing herpes at the end of a year. It's not zero, because condoms don't cover all the areas where the virus can be spread. Just so you know, though, an uninfected woman is at higher risk of getting herpes from an infected male than vice versa," rattled off Dr. Dylan.

"Why's that?"

"During sex, a woman gets microscopic abrasions in her vagina that make her more susceptible to disease. By the way, from your question, I'm assuming your new girlfriend doesn't have genital herpes. Do you know if she gets the mouth sores of oral herpes?" asked Dr. Dylan.

"I've never seen one on her, but to be honest, we haven't had a discussion about it yet. Does it matter?" wondered Justin.

"Yes, actually, it does. If she already has oral herpes, that ten percent risk number I told you is accurate. If, however, she doesn't have antibodies to any type of herpes, her chance of getting herpes from you goes up to about thirty-two percent."

"So you're basically telling me that I should actually hope that Kayla has oral herpes. Great. That's what got me into this in the first place. What about beyond a year? Just for the sake of discussion, say we got married, for example. Is she guaranteed to get herpes from me? Obviously, if we wanted to have kids, we wouldn't be using a condom then," said Justin.

"Well, there are some long-term couples in which one partner has herpes, and the other one seems to be free of disease. Perhaps they have a mild case that they're unaware of, or they just have great antibodies. Either way, it does happen, but we don't have enough long-term studies to give you a solid answer right now.

"What you really need to know is that you are contagious, whether or not you have an outbreak. You definitely shed more virus immediately before, during, and after an outbreak, but it's thought that up to seventy percent of transmission occurs when people think they are not contagious," Dr. Dylan lectured.

"That doesn't make sense," muttered Justin, doing the math in his head.

"Think about it," said Dr. Dylan. "People are more careful, abstaining from sex when they feel symptoms like burning or itching before an outbreak, and certainly when they can see blisters, right? And that's when they shed the most virus so potentially are the most contagious."

"Okay," agreed Justin.

"But in between outbreaks, when there is no visible sign of herpes, so people don't feel contagious, they are intimate more often. So they are less contagious, but more sexually active, and therefore, more infections are transmitted," clarified the doctor.

"Well, I saw on a commercial that if you take this medicine every day, it's supposed to help decrease the chance that you can pass on the infection. Is that true?" inquired Justin.

"Yes, fortunately, it is. Studies have proven that if you take suppressive daily valacyclovir, a herpes antiviral drug, it decreases the risk of passing on herpes to an uninfected partner by up to fifty percent."

"What about hot tubs? If I'm having an outbreak, so I'm shedding all this virus, can I give it to people if we all go hot-tubbing together?" asked Justin.

Dr. Dylan laughed. "No. Don't be concerned about that. No hot tubs, toilet seats, or any other objects that people share purely externally can transmit the virus. This virus is not that hardy. It dies when the secretions carrying it dry up. Now, two people sharing sex toys could absolutely pass it on, but just hanging around other people is perfectly safe."

"No worries there," Justin replied. He sat for a moment, processing everything the doctor had said.

Dr. Dylan stood up, handing Justin the prescription. "Here you go. Let me examine you quickly to make sure this is genital herpes. I know we've confirmed it before, so I was assuming you were pretty sure about the diagnosis. Have you had any new sexual partners since your last visit?"

It was Justin's turn to laugh. "No, Dr. Dylan. I've actually never even had sex. I got this from my high school girlfriend from having oral sex a few times. I can't imagine what else this could be—it's a clump of small blisters in the same spot where they always show up."

Dr. Dylan motioned for Justin to lie back. "Let's just take a look to be sure." It took only a few seconds, and then Dr. Dylan's confirmation came with a more sympathetic tone. "Yes, Justin, this a very typical lesion. See here, the base is bright red, and your cluster of blisters is already scabbing over." He sat down on his stool and flipped back through Justin's chart again.

"What are you looking for?" asked Justin.

"Well, I'm looking to see if we ever checked your antibodies to see what type of herpes you have. Classically, herpes type one used to be the main source of oral herpes, and type two was the cause of genital lesions, but now it's closer to an equal distribution."

"What difference does it make?" wondered Justin.

"I guess it's a bit academic," said Dr. Dylan, "but usually type one herpes in the genital region doesn't cause as many outbreaks as you've dealt with, so I was curious." He paused for a moment, then added, "Also, I was thinking about your new girlfriend. If you know what type of herpes you have, she can be tested to see if she has antibodies. Most adults have antibodies to at least one type of herpes, and if she has antibodies to the same type that you have, she'll be somewhat protected."

A wave of cautious optimism began to creep over Justin. "Okay, then, if it's not in my chart, let's test me and find out. I don't remember anyone ever telling me which type. I thought since it was in my crotch, I automatically had type two. I never thought about where it came from. So, if you have type one, for example, you can still catch type two, but it doesn't matter where in your body you or the other person has herpes. Is that right?"

Dr. Dylan nodded. "That's more or less correct. You contract herpes only by direct contact with it, so in that sense, it does matter where you or your partner have it. Typically, a person infected with one type of herpes in their genitals will not get a new genital infection of herpes simplex virus, or HSV, even if they are exposed to a different type. Also, if you have type one herpes in your genital area, and your girlfriend has type one herpes in her mouth, you will not develop a new spot of herpes if she performs oral sex on you. Does that make sense?"

Justin nodded in agreement, still absorbing the information.

Dr. Dylan continued, "However, if you have type one genital herpes, and she has type two oral herpes, you potentially could catch a new infection. The most likely place for it to show up, though, would be in your mouth, from kissing her."

"And if, instead, I have type two down there?" quizzed Justin.

"Type two herpes seems to produce a much more protective antibody response. If you have type two herpes in your genitals, you are usually protected against developing a new type one infection anywhere in your body," said Dr. Dylan.

"Usually, meaning not one hundred percent, I'm assuming," interrupted Justin.

"Yes. Of course, no matter what, I recommend using a condom if you're having any kind of sex, to prevent not only spreading herpes but any other disease as well. If you're thinking about having sex with your girlfriend, I'd advise that both of you be fully tested for all sexually transmitted diseases. We can add that today, if you'd like," advised Dr. Dylan.

"What else could I possibly have, if I've never had real sex?" asked Justin.

"Well, we know you've had enough exposure to get herpes, which means you could potentially have another disease. It sounds like you are certainly at a lower risk, but it's not zero. I'd still just check you for everything, including gonorrhea, chlamydia, HIV, hepatitis C, and syphilis. You're immunized against hepatitis B, so at least we don't need to worry about that one. I didn't see any genital warts, lice, or other obvious lesions. Look, it's far easier to have an honest conversation with your girlfriend if you can assure one another that you have truly been tested for all sexually transmittable diseases." Dr. Dylan stood up, handing Justin his lab slip. "Most diseases are not as obvious as your herpes. Lots of them don't even have any symptoms. If you are going to be sexually intimate, whether you think it's 'real sex' or not, wear condoms every time, and talk to your partner about all this before you're in a situation where talking isn't your priority. I gave you a three-month supply of valacyclovir, or Valtrex. Why don't you follow up with me at the end of the prescription and let me know if it stopped the outbreaks, okay?"

Justin went to the lab and had his blood drawn, then stopped at the pharmacy to get his medicine. He still wasn't positive how long he was going to take it, but it seemed reasonable enough to give it a try.

A few days went by, and Justin had no side effects that he was aware of from the medicine. His lesions had cleared up enough that he felt okay to bike ride again, so he suggested an Italian café for their Friday night dinner.

"Gotta love carbo-loading," murmured Justin, swallowing a mouthful of pasta.

"Where do you want to ride tomorrow?" asked Kayla, wiping her mouth free of sauce. She grimaced when she touched the corner of her mouth. "Oh man, I think I'm getting another cold sore," she complained.

Startled, Justin leaned forward across the table, staring intently at her mouth. "Do you have herpes?" he blurted out. He was partly dismayed, but at the same time partly relieved.

Kayla pulled back, her hand protectively covering her mouth. "Yuck—herpes?" her face contorted in an appalled look. "No! I just get mouth ulcers when I'm stressed out. With finals around the corner, I'm not surprised if I'm getting one. What makes you think it's herpes? Do you have herpes?" she blurted.

Here it was, the moment of truth. But the look of disgust on Kayla's face as she said "herpes" was too much. If Kayla thought a mouth ulcer was "yucky," what would she think if he told her he had sores in his crotch? Justin's brain raced wildly, wanting to be honest but fearful it was too early in their relationship to broach the whole topic.

"No, I don't get mouth sores," Justin said, skirting around the complete truth. "It's no big deal anyway, I was just curious. I read somewhere that most mouth ulcers were herpes. You see those commercials on television all the time now, so I was just going to say you might want to check with your doctor to see if one could help you." Quickly, he switched topics. "Anyway, back to the ride. I thought maybe we'd head over to Bastrop and bike in the pine woods tomorrow. I hear there are some great hills to conquer over there, if you're up for it," he challenged.

"Bet I can beat you up the last hill," Kayla retorted, and happily chatted on about the weather expected in the morning.

Justin realized this conversation might come back to haunt him some day, but technically, he had been honest. At least he knew there was a strong chance that she already had one type of herpes, and there was a fifty percent chance that it would be the same type as his. Justin's testing had shown that he had type two herpes simplex, which explained his frequent outbreaks. The doctor felt that the overall health benefits of Justin's biking outweighed the down side of it possibly triggering frequent HSV recurrences. Justin promised himself that the next time the subject came up, he would tell Kayla the story of his high school girlfriend and how he got herpes.

For now, he'd be content to get to know Kayla better, and perhaps learn more about her past experiences. Justin glanced at her mouth again, only barely able to see the sore that was forming just above the corner of her mouth. He remembered that his type two infection would primarily protect him against a new type two infection, and that Kayla's presumed oral herpes could be either type. "Better not do any kissing tonight," he thought, startling himself with what seemed a bit of a double standard.

"Really," Justin thought, "just because I don't want to get oral herpes, I'm not being unreasonable, now that I understand about the different types." But the more he pondered it, the more he was sincerely worried about catching oral herpes. Justin knew that he couldn't go back to kissing Kayla until they knew which type she had, which meant having a full-blown conversation about sexually transmittable diseases.

"Hey, there, are you listening? I was asking if you wanted a taste of my tiramisu?" Kayla interrupted his internal debate as she extended a piece of her dessert on a fork.

Justin internally recoiled, but he simply said, "No thanks, I'm too stuffed to manage even one more bite." "Oh well," he thought to himself, "I guess we'll have a lot to talk about on our ride tomorrow."

facts

Herpes Simplex Virus (HSV) Fact Sheet

What is it?

- Herpes is a DNA virus.

- There are two strains: type 1 and type 2.

- Type 1 more commonly occurs in the mouth, and type 2 more often in the genitals, but both can occur in either location.

- One person can be infected with both types.

How common is it?

- Estimates vary, but between 50 and 90% of adults have oral herpes by age 50.

- 25% of adults have genital herpes, but up to 90% of them are unaware of it.

How do you get it?

- Through direct skin contact with an infected area.

- From secretions infected with HSV: saliva, vaginal secretions, or semen (including on shared utensils or toothbrushes).

Where on your body do you get it?

- Most often in a mucosal surface: mouth or genital skin.

- Less often on any skin surface, such as arms or legs, unless skin is broken (for example, if it has been bitten or scratched).

How do I know if I have it?

- Many people are asymptomatic, so the only way to know if you have been infected is to check blood tests.

- Blood tests check for antibodies to HSV1 and HSV2.

- HSV DNA testing or a herpes culture taken by swabbing a new lesion can confirm herpes infection.

What does it look like?

- A small red bump or blister or cluster of bumps or blisters on a bright red base.

What does it feel like?

- Many people feel itching, burning, or tingling before they see any lesions.

- Blisters may be extremely painful or mildly annoying.

- Nearby lymph nodes (in neck or groin) may swell and ache.

- Especially with the initial outbreak, additional symptoms may include headache, muscle aches, stiff neck, sore throat, fever, and flu-like symptoms.

How long does it last?

- Initial outbreak lasts 1–2 weeks on average.

- Recurrent outbreaks last 3–7 days.

Can it be cured?

- No. Once infected, you will always have the virus.

What is the treatment?

- Antiviral medicines such as acyclovir (Zovirax), famciclovir (Famvir), and valacyclovir (Valtrex) can reduce the duration and intensity of an outbreak if taken as soon as you are aware of symptoms, preferably before blisters even form.

- Medicines can be taken daily to prevent frequent recurrences.

How about alternative therapies?

- Wearing loose clothes can allow the sores to dry out.

- Reducing stress can help prevent breakouts.

- Some patients may find taking daily lysine supplements decreases the frequency or intensity of breakouts, but there are no large clinical studies confirming this practice.

Are there long-term consequences of herpes?

- HSV does not cause scarring unless there is a secondary infection from a bacteria (like a staph or strep infection caused by scratching).

- New HSV infections during pregnancy are harmful to the fetus, and HSV can infect a child passing through the birth canal. Most expectant mothers who have herpes choose to have a Cesarean section to decrease risk of transmission.

When are you contagious?

- Always!

- Herpes is most infective immediately before, during, and after an outbreak.

How do I avoid getting genital herpes?

- Abstinence from sexual intimacy (direct genital contact; oral, vaginal, and/or anal sex) is the only 100% effective prevention.

- Condom use decreases transmission but is not totally effective because virus can be shed outside of the area that condoms cover.

- Use new condoms for each partner with any shared sex toys, or preferably, do not share sex toys.

If I have herpes, how do I avoid giving it to my partner?

- Daily valacyclovir (suppressive treatment) can reduce viral shedding and therefore reduce transmission of herpes.

- Abstinence during outbreaks paired with condom use in

between outbreaks reduces the transmission of herpes to an uninfected partner.

Does herpes transmission occur in homosexual partners?

- Oral-genital transmission can occur regardless of gender.

- Shared sex toys can transmit the herpes virus.

- Herpes can be transmitted during anal intercourse.

Frequently Asked Questions

➤ **Can you catch herpes from a toilet seat?**
No. The virus dies quickly outside the body, especially when it gets dry.

➤ **Are most oral "cold sores" from vitamin deficiencies?**
No. Most cold sores are herpes simplex.

➤ **Can you catch genital herpes from oral sex?**
Yes. This is a frequent source of transmission.

➤ **If you can't see or feel any sores, are you contagious?**
Yes. If you have herpes, you are always potentially contagious.

➤ **If you develop herpes in a monogamous relationship, is your partner cheating?**
Not necessarily, because it can take weeks, months, or years after exposure until you first notice an outbreak.

Additional Information

American College of Obstetricians and Gynecologists
P. O. Box 96920
409 12th Street, SW
Washington, DC 20090-6920
202-863-2518
www.acog.org/publications/patient_education/bp054.cfm

CDC-INFO
Centers for Disease Control and Prevention
1600 Clifton Road
Atlanta, GA 30333
1-800-CDC-INFO (1-800-232-4636), 1-888-232-6348 TTY
www.cdc.gov/std/Herpes/default.htm

MedlinePlus
National Library of Medicine
8600 Rockville Pike
Bethesda, MD 20894
1-888-FIND-NLM (1-888-346-3656), or 301-594-5983
www.nlm.nih.gov/medlineplus/herpessimplex.html

National Herpes Resource Center and Hotline
American Social Health Association
P. O. Box 13827
Research Triangle Park, NC 27709
919-361-8488 (9 a.m. to 7 p.m. EST, Mon. through Fri.)
www.ashastd.org/hrc/index.html

HUMAN PAPILLOMA VIRUS

3: Chad

CHAD GLANCED AROUND the waiting room. Here and there, people smiled and nodded at him with recognition. At six foot four, 210 pounds, with bright red hair and freckles, Chad tended to stick out in a crowd. Oh great, he thought. Of all the times to be recognized, this was not the right one. This year had been absolutely amazing so far. Here it was, his senior year of high school, and he was picked over his long-term rival and buddy, Frank, to be the first-string quarterback. Although the first couple of games had been a bit shaky, by the third game he had found his groove and the Chargers were easily dominating their opponents each week. His picture had been plastered across the front page of the local paper, and now everyone was speculating about which college recruiters were after him.

"I think they know my football star son," Chad's mother whispered to him with pride. Chad groaned in response. His mom continued, "Don't worry, I'm sure Dr. Morris will get you fixed up in time for this Friday, honey. Can you believe the scouts from UCLA are coming to the game?" Chad's mom was a UCLA alumna, and she would love nothing more than to see her son playing for her alma mater. "Besides, Dr. Morris is a Bruin, too, so I know she'll want you in top form this weekend. Do you think she'll be wearing her blue-and-gold scrubs today?"

Chad smiled. He'd been seeing Dr. Morris since grade school. He had outgrown the sticker and lollipop rewards at the end of the visits, but he still enjoyed seeing her. Dr. Morris bounded with energy and always made him laugh. Most of her staff supported the other local university and football powerhouse, the USC Trojans, but Dr. Morris was always optimistic that her Bruins would some day win the national championship. She had teased Chad for years that he would be just the quarterback to lead them to that victory.

Shifting nervously in his chair, Chad thought about explaining today's visit to the doctor. He must have made a face, because suddenly his mom's brow furrowed, and she asked him, "Does it hurt very much? I hope that giving you ibuprofen was the right thing to do."

"Honestly, it's really not that bad anymore, Mom," Chad said. "I mainly just want to be sure that I'm in good shape this week. I bet I won't even have to miss a practice."

"Chad?" Alice, the nurse, stood at the door to the office and called out his name from the chart she held in her hands. Chad jumped up, waving his mom back.

"Uh, Mom, I'm fine by myself. Just wait out here, and I'll be right back." Chad's mom was already half out of her chair, ready to follow him back.

"Okay, honey. If you'd rather see the doctor by yourself, I guess I'll wait here," she said with a martyred sigh. Chad let out his own sigh, one of relief, and was thankful that he had begun occasionally seeing Dr. Morris by himself a few years ago. Now his mom wouldn't be suspicious that anything was up.

His mother had insisted on driving him this morning, claiming her parental rights since he was leaving for college in six months, and saying that she had a right to baby him as long as he lived at home. His dad had even offered to bring him, but Chad had quickly reassured both of them that the whole office visit was just a precaution. The nurse walked him down the familiar hallway, stopping at the scale to weigh him.

"That was some game you played Friday night," she said with a warm smile. "You're giving those cheerleaders lots of reasons to celebrate this year."

Chad grinned, saying, "Let's hope we do it again this weekend. This game will be much tougher."

"Well, then we'll just have to make sure we've got you in perfect health by then. No pressure, after all, we've got four whole days 'til the next game." They both laughed as she led him into an exam room and motioned for him to sit on the exam table.

"Okay, Chad," Alice said as she wrapped the blood pressure cuff around his arm, "so you pulled something in your groin Friday night?"

"Um, I guess that's what happened..." Chad's voice trailed off. At what point did he need to tell the truth? Did it matter what he said to the nurse, or could he just wait until Dr. Morris came in?

"How did it happen? Did it start hurting immediately after you were tackled, or did you not notice it until after the game?" Chad felt his face flushing.

"Uh...to be honest...I was embarrassed to tell the receptionist, but..." he bit his lip and swallowed hard.

"Chad." He looked up at the nurse. Alice had worked at Dr. Morris's office since Chad started middle school. She smiled gently, removing the cuff from his arm.

"Don't worry, if there is something else you need to tell the doctor, remember we're here to take care of any problem you have—even if it's embarrassing. Do you feel comfortable telling me what's really going on?" Chad wanted to just disappear. He tried to act like he was talking about something completely boring.

"Well," he said, willing his voice to jump back down to the right octave, "I'm sure it's nothing, but I noticed a few bumps on my...uh...down there." He pointed at his crotch. "It seems like they're kind of multiplying, so I thought I'd better get it checked out. It's probably from my jock strap, or something." His voice trailed off.

"It's okay, Chad, Dr. Morris will figure out what's going on, and she'll help you fix it. Please go ahead and get undressed from the waist down, and you can put this sheet over yourself and sit on the end of the exam table. Dr. Morris will be in shortly." She handed him the sheet, grabbed his chart and stepped out of the room.

Chad quickly shed his jeans and boxers and situated himself on the end of the table. He thought back to Saturday morning. He had been going through his usual postgame Saturday morning routine of soaking in a hot bath and letting his stiff muscles begin to relax, when he saw the bumps. A few weeks ago, he had noticed two small reddish bumps just below the head of his penis. They didn't itch or hurt, and he basically had ignored them and figured they would go away. Last weekend though, he was dismayed to see that there seemed to be a whole cluster of them, and they looked kind of wrinkly on top. Chad knew he had to go see Dr. Morris and find out what was going on.

However, there was no way that he would tell his parents there was something growing on his penis. "Can you imagine what a tirade of questions that would set off?" Chad thought. His dad already was giving him monthly speeches about the "birds and the bees," which basically consisted of his dad stammering around for awhile and ending up saying, "Son, just be sure you use condoms. You don't want to get some girl pregnant and ruin both of your lives, not to mention your football career. Remember, sports are your ticket to a college education, and education"—here Chad would join in and finish the sentence—"is your ticket to life." His parents pretty much stayed out of his social life, though his mom had asked a bunch of questions when he and Vanessa started hanging out together last summer.

Vanessa babysat for her next-door neighbor's kids in the mornings. Chad and a few of his buddies mowed lawns, but they usually tried to finish their work by noon, before it got too hot. This left their afternoons free, and a big group got together most afternoons and evenings at the lake. Vanessa's parents had a lake house with a boat, so that was the usual gathering place. They loved skiing, wakeboarding, and just hanging out. Their friends were mainly jocks and cheerleaders, all of them filled with anticipation for their senior year. Within the group, there were several couples that were "serious."

By midsummer, Chad was having sex with Vanessa. Chad knew enough to use condoms, even though she was on the pill. Her parents thought she was taking the pill just to help with her periods, and she told Chad that she was a virgin. They pledged their love to one another and talked of going off to the same college. In fairness, Chad thought now, she had talked much more about their future together, and he was more excited about the present.

At any rate, Chad's parents had seemed relieved when he and Vanessa broke up in August. They liked her well enough, but his mom was convinced that Vanessa was trying to tie him down, and his dad was mainly worried that she would distract him from football practice. The truth was, when Vanessa dumped Chad in August for another guy, he was devastated. It was, however, great motivation for him during the hot two-a-day practices. He was so bummed out and jealous of Vanessa's new boyfriend that he threw his heart and soul into practices, taking out all his aggressions on the practice field.

By October, Vanessa had broken up with the new guy and was giving Chad big smiles and major hints that she was free again. At an after-game celebration, Chad's resolve to make her wait completely melted when she bounded up and hugged him. A quick kiss turned into a late-night makeout session, and before he knew it, they were right back where they had left off. That first night, he wasn't prepared with condoms. On the exam table, as he contemplated the cluster of bumps on his genitals, he thought back to that hasty decision.

Luckily, Chad didn't have to wait very long for the doctor. He heard a knock, followed by Dr. Morris's voice asking, "Ready?" as she came in and sat on her stool. The nurse, who had followed her in, went over to the corner behind Chad and was busily setting something out on the countertops. Chad knew that it was the policy of this office to have a nurse "chaperone" any time a patient's "private parts" were examined. He remembered his initial embarrassment during his annual checkups when Dr. Morris taught him how to perform a testicular self-exam for cancer and when she did the dreaded "turn your head and cough" check for a hernia. Over the years, his comfort level had increased to where he barely even noticed the nurse, but today he was just embarrassed to have anyone other than Dr. Morris around to see this.

"Okay, Chad, so you've got some bumps?" the doctor asked. Suddenly, his mouth went dry, and he couldn't speak. He nodded his head yes. He was relieved that, as usual, she cut to the chase. "Well, when did you first notice them?"

"About three weeks ago," he managed to croak.

"Do they hurt?"

Good, a yes/no question, he thought. "No."

"Itch?"

"No."

"But they're getting worse?"

Chad swallowed hard and made eye contact with Dr. Morris. "Um, yeah. There are more of them."

"Have you had sex?" she asked. Now he was really squirming. How many times had she talked to him about using condoms?

"Yes." He knew what was coming next.

"And did you use condoms?"

He couldn't look up any longer. "Mostly," he managed to stammer.

Dr. Morris half smiled and raised her right eyebrow. "'Mostly,' meaning there were times that you had sex that you did not wear a condom?"

"Uh, right," confessed Chad.

"Well, Chad, with skin things, a picture's often worth a thousand words. Let's take a look and see what we're talking about." She put on a pair of gloves and reached down to slide out the bottom section of the table so he could fit on the table with his feet extended. "Go ahead and lie back," she said. She lifted the drape and began examining his bumps.

"So, uh, Dr. Morris, do you think it could just be a rash from my jock strap?" he asked hopefully.

"I'm sorry, Chad, but I don't think so. Sit up for a second and look here at the tops of the bumps. Do you see how wrinkly they look? These are warts."

WARTS? His stomach sunk. Geez, his worst fears were right. He hadn't realized how much he was counting on those fears being wrong.

"Okay, Chad, why don't you go ahead and sit up. We need to talk about treatment."

Chad sat up, still freaking out about having warts. A venereal disease—gross. They had seen pictures in their health class, but then everyone had just laughed and made jokes about "VDs." It wasn't funny at all when it's you with the disease. What was Vanessa going to think? Suddenly, it hit him. Vanessa. Why was he worried about what she thought? It had to be her that had given it to him. She must have slept with that jerk when they broke up last summer.

"Chad? Are you listening?" Dr. Morris asked.

"I'm sorry, Dr. Morris, I was just wondering how I got these. I mean, I know how I got them, but..."

"It's okay. Let's talk about treatment first, and then after you get dressed, I will tell you everything you need to know about warts, including what you need to tell your girlfriend."

"There are several methods used to treat genital warts. We can use topical acids to burn them, or liquid nitrogen to freeze them. For yours, I think we should use the liquid nitrogen. We can do that right now, in a matter of minutes. You know I'm always honest with you, Chad, so I will tell you that it is going to hurt. It burns pretty badly for about thirty seconds, but then it will just ache. The problem for you is that after we treat them, the area will blister up, get red, and swell for five to seven days. It will definitely be uncomfortable for you, especially in a jock strap. We could wait until after football season to treat them, but they could grow and multiply quite a bit in the next couple of months, so that would not be my recommendation. The smaller these are and the fewer you have, the easier it is to treat them. However, it's your call. I realize this could affect your practice this week. What do you think?"

Chad was still just trying to grasp the fact that he had warts—genital warts. He shook his head, trying unsuccessfully to clear his thoughts. "Okay, if I do it now, how much do you think it will bug me at practice? I really just want to get rid of them."

"Well, typically they bother patients the most during the first few days. It's just hard to say, because wearing football gear might aggravate it and delay healing a bit. Honestly, I think you'll be fine, but everyone reacts differently to the freezing, so it's truly hard to predict." Chad knew there was no way he could just delay treatment until December. He felt so gross to have warts down there. There was only one decision.

"Let's just treat them now and get it over with. They won't come back, will they?" He looked expectantly at the doctor. Unfortunately, there was no smile now. Dr. Morris looked him right in the eyes.

"Chad, warts are caused by a virus—the human papilloma virus, or HPV for short. There are many different strains, but the thing they all share in common is that we do not yet have a cure for warts. We can treat outbreaks, but we cannot kill the virus."

Chad's mouth dropped open in disbelief. "You're telling me that I'm going to have this the rest of my life?"

"Well, right now we do not have a cure, so the answer today is yes, you will carry the virus the rest of your life. It does not mean that you will always have actual warts growing. Anyway, let's go ahead and treat the ones you've got now, and then after you're dressed, I promise to answer all your questions, okay?" Chad nodded yes, and lay back on the exam table, closing his eyes.

During this conversation, the nurse had discreetly slipped out of the room, and now she popped back in with a silver canister. "Chad, this is liquid nitrogen," Dr. Morris said. "I'm going to spray it on each wart until it makes a little frozen ball on top, then after they thaw in a few seconds, we repeat that sequence a few times. It will sting and burn while I do this, but it shouldn't last more than five minutes or so to treat all of them. Are you ready?"

Chad felt his heart racing with anxiety as he replied, "Ready as I'll ever be. Go ahead." He watched with a detached fascination as she sprayed each wart. Then came the pain. He gritted his teeth as it began to feel like a bee was stinging him. This would be bad enough for a wart on a finger or a knee, but on his penis? How could this have happened to him?

"Okay, last round. Are you hanging in there?" asked Dr. Morris.

"Yeah. You weren't kidding when you said this would hurt, though."

Dr. Morris smiled. "You know me, Chad. I always tell the truth. I never tell kids shots don't hurt, so I wouldn't lie about this stinging. Ready?"

"Okay. Tell me when you're done." Chad closed his eyes again and started counting. He figured that if he could focus on counting, she should be finished by the time he got to one hundred. As it turned out, he only had to count to thirty-two.

"Okay, we're done. Alice is going to put some ointment on it, and then you can get dressed. I'll come back in a minute and bring you more information about warts."

With that, the doctor left the room, and the nurse began smoothing on some ointment.

"This has a little bit of topical anesthetic in it along with the antibiotic, so it should help with the discomfort. Is the stinging going away yet?" asked Alice.

Chad was just relieved the procedure was finished. "To be honest, it still burns, but not as bad as when she was spraying that stuff on there."

"Well, it will get better throughout the day. Go ahead and shower normally, cleaning the area with your regular soap and water. The skin is going to blister up and get red before the warts go away. See how it's already swollen?"

Chad looked at his crotch. Everywhere the spray had touched was now bright red and starting to swell. Man, I sure hope no one notices this in the showers after practice, he thought.

"Give yourself a minute when you sit up before you get dressed," said Alice. "You might feel a bit light-headed." Then Alice left the room, and Chad was alone.

He felt tears welling up in his eyes. How could he have warts? The question kept circling around in his brain. Because you had sex without a condom, you idiot, came the answer. What was he going to say to Vanessa? He must have gotten it from her. Did she know she had warts? He certainly had never seen any on her, not that he'd exactly ever been looking, now that he thought about it. "For the rest of your life," the doctor had said. Man, he was only eighteen.

Knock, knock. "Ready?" In came Dr. Morris. Chad was back in his jeans and sitting up on the exam table.

"I'm sure you've got a lot of questions for me, Chad. I brought you some handouts on the wart virus for you to take home and read later, but let's talk about some basics now. Warts are a sexually transmitted disease, as I'm sure you know. Many people carry the wart virus without realizing that they are infected. Women can actually have warts internally, inside their vaginas, and not be able to see them. Oftentimes the only way women know that they carry the virus is through an abnormal Pap smear, which is a screening test for cervical cancer that they get at their annual gynecological exams. Obviously, you need to talk with anyone you've had sex with. Have you had more than one partner?"

"I had sex once a year ago with someone else, but I've only been with my girlfriend, Vanessa, in the past six months."

"Well, technically, it's possible that you could have received the virus from either girl, then, but given the timing, it's more likely that it came from Vanessa. You'll need to tell her and encourage her to go and get examined and get a Pap smear."

"Why does she need the Pap smear? Didn't you just say that it is a test for cancer?" asked Chad.

"Yes, it is," replied Dr. Morris, "but the Pap test can also potentially detect the presence of the wart virus. In fact, the worst thing about the wart virus is that some strains of it can lead to cervical cancer in women, although the two strains of the wart virus that cause ninety percent of genital warts do not typically lead to cancer. If Vanessa's Pap test shows any wart virus, further testing can determine if she has one of the strains that place her at high risk for developing cervical cancer. Virtually all cervical cancers are caused by the papilloma virus, which makes cervical cancer effectively a sexually transmitted disease.

"Anyway, you need to know that even when you don't have any visible warts, you can still pass on the virus. So ultimately, you absolutely need to use condoms any time that you have sex from now on, and even then, you really need to tell the woman that you're a carrier of the virus, since condoms are not foolproof."

"Honestly, right now, the thought of ever having sex with anyone again is the last thing on my mind," said Chad.

Dr. Morris smiled. "I certainly can understand that, but the truth is that you are young, and chances are that you will, so I want you to have all the information that you need. Do you have any other questions right now?" Chad thought for a minute. It was hard to digest all this information at once. He glanced at the brochures in his hands. "No, I'm sure these will cover any other questions that I have."

All of a sudden, he remembered his mom was waiting in the waiting area. What was he going to tell her?

"Wait. I do have a question," he said quickly.

Dr. Morris sat back down. "Fire away," she said.

"Um, my mom is here. Do we have to tell her about this?"

Dr. Morris sighed. "Chad, to be honest, I would recommend that you do tell her. You are eighteen, which means that we do not have to tell her anything about your medical care. However, on the bill, under the procedure codes, it's going to say that we treated some warts, so your mom will find that out when she gets the bill from the insurance company."

"Can't you just put something else down for the bill?" Chad almost begged.

"No, I'm sorry, I really can't, because that's insurance fraud. That would get me in trouble. It's your decision what you tell her, though. It doesn't specify genital warts."

"So I could say that I had a groin pull, but that you also treated a wart somewhere else, like on my leg or something?" he pleaded.

"That would be your choice. Chad, if your mom asks me a question directly, I won't lie. Now that you're eighteen I am legally obligated to tell her that I cannot talk to her without your permission, but I won't make anything up to cover, or tell her anything that's not true. Actually, here in California and in most states, since this is a sexually transmittable disease, you would have the right to decide about your treatment regardless of your age, without the knowledge or consent of your parents."

Chad felt miserable. He could just see the look of shock and disappointment and the tears that were sure to come if his mom found out the truth. Not to mention his dad—Chad couldn't even imagine his response. "I understand. You've always treated me right, and I don't want to get you in trouble for my screwup. I...I just don't think I can tell her today, Dr. Morris. I promise to come up with a way to talk to her about this before she hears anything from the insurance company."

Chad stood up and shook the doctor's hand. "Thanks a lot. I'll read this stuff, and I swear I'll be more careful in the future," he said.

"I'm sure you will, Chad. Come back and see me in a couple of weeks if the warts don't completely go away with this treatment. Otherwise, I'll just see you back for your checkup before you leave for college, okay? And feel free to call with any questions that come up that aren't answered in those handouts." They stepped out of the room, and Chad began to walk down the hallway.

"Oh, Chad—one more thing." Chad spun around, wondering what she could have forgotten to tell him. Dr. Morris just grinned and added, "Knock 'em dead this season."

Chad had to smile. If only everything were as easy as football.

4: Heather

HEATHER CLOSED HER EYES on the dance floor, tossing her curly black hair with the beat. Scott was admiring her long athletic legs and tight black miniskirt. Her stiletto heels only brought Heather up to Scott's chest. Scott's six-foot-six frame gave him a natural advantage on Tech's track team, for which he ran cross-country. As the packed crowd swayed and shoved Scott awkwardly into Heather yet again, he decided he'd had enough dancing. "Come on," he said to her, "Let's take a break and grab something to drink."

Scott grabbed Heather's hand, and her heart soared as she followed him, looking around the crowded bar to see if any of her friends saw her holding hands with Scott. Heather's first year at Tech had been filled with dates, but she had been hoping to go out with Scott since she met him at a dorm mixer at the beginning of the year. He literally stood out in a crowd, towering above most of his classmates.

Scott and Heather shared the same biology class, along with a couple hundred other freshmen, but both of them liked to sit in the back row, right by the doors. Heather thought it was funny how everyone tended to sit in the same spot, as though there were assigned seating in the huge auditorium. That tendency allowed her to get to know the small group of students who sat in her area, including Scott. He had never asked her out, but tonight when they ran into each other at the club, Scott finally seemed interested. Heather had actually asked him to dance, but now here he was, gripping her hand and smiling down at her.

"What do you want to drink?" shouted Scott over the music.

"Diet Coke," Heather shouted back.

Scott ordered their drinks and a basket of chips, and then lunged for a nearby table that had just opened up. Heather happily slid into the chair that Scott held out.

"Great job snagging a table," she complimented, reaching down to rub her aching feet.

"I hope I'm not the reason your feet hurt," said Scott sheepishly. "I know I must have stepped on your toes more than once out there."

"No, really, it's just the high heels," laughed Heather. "I'm far more comfortable in my sneakers, but they didn't quite go with this outfit."

Scott smiled at this mental image of Heather in her sexy top and short skirt paired with tennis shoes. "I don't know why not. At least you'd be more comfortable. Anyway, you look great. You should wear this outfit to our biology class," he joked.

"Thanks, maybe I will. Are you ready for the test next Friday?" Heather asked.

"Not yet. Why don't we grab dinner next Thursday, and we can study together afterwards?" Scott asked smoothly.

"Sure, that sounds great," Heather smiled, as she inwardly jumped up and down. Their conversation flowed easily as they polished off their chips and sodas. Too soon, Scott's roommate, Steve, rushed up, grabbing Scott by the arm.

"Come on, Scott. Sorry to interrupt, but really, we were supposed to be at Suzy's party an hour ago. I've been looking all over for you." Steve gave Heather an apologetic look and added, "Suzy's my girlfriend. She's going to kill me if we're any later."

"Sorry, Heather, but I really do have to go. It was my turn to drive tonight, and we promised Suzy we were just stopping by here for a few minutes." Scott stood to go. "We're on for next Thursday, though, right?"

"It's a date," Heather agreed with a smile. She watched the two guys head out of the club, then searched for her friends to share the news. She found Amelia and Kate in the bathroom, touching up their lipstick and hair.

"You did it," squealed Amelia.

"Scott is so cute," gushed Kate. "I'm so proud of you for asking him to dance. You guys were out there a long time."

"And I saw you over in the corner at a table," added Amelia. "So, tell us everything."

"He actually asked me out!" Heather recounted her conversation with Scott, and the girls' chatter continued as Heather went into the stall. When she wiped herself, she was surprised to see a bit of blood on the toilet paper. "Hey, does anyone have a tampon with them? I can't believe my period just started. It's not due for another week or so," Heather complained. Unfortunately, her friends had only brought their driver's licenses, money, and lipstick to the club, and naturally the machine in the bathroom was out of feminine hygiene products.

"Oh well, no big deal. I'm going to head back to the dorm and call it a night," Heather said as the girls left the bathroom.

"At least you don't have to just dream about Scott any more," Amelia said encouragingly. "You can look forward to next week. Kate and I have got to get back out on that dance floor and see if we can meet some decent guys. Wish us luck."

Heather headed back to her dorm, caught up again in the excitement of her evening. As she showered, she felt a couple of small bumps below her vagina. When she got out and toweled off, there was another spot of blood, so she tried to look in the mirror to figure out where the spotting was coming from. It was an incredibly awkward position, so Heather couldn't see well enough to be sure, but it looked like the spots of blood were coming from her rectum, not from a period starting early. She got dressed and went to her computer.

"Okay, what the heck do I call this?" Heather wondered, as she pulled up her favorite search engine. "How about rectal bleeding?" Links to more than a million sites popped up. "Oh brother," she thought to herself, but clicked on the two or three sites that looked the most official. Heather read through the descriptions, and because she had no history of abdominal cramps or diarrhea, she assumed she had developed hemorrhoids. "Wow, age eighteen, and I've already got an old lady's disease," Heather thought. She'd overheard some of her mom's friends complaining about hemorrhoids after having babies. Heather entered "hemorrhoids" in her search engine, then chose the Mayo Clinic website, figuring that it must be reliable. This site cautioned that while hemorrhoids are common, if a person has new rectal bleeding, a doctor should determine the cause. Heather decided she would call for an appointment the next week if the spotting continued, then logged off her computer and climbed into bed, not thinking at all about rectal bleeding but happily replaying the evening in her head.

Several weeks went by, and Heather had more or less forgotten about the whole bleeding episode. No pain or cramps, and she hadn't noticed any new spotting. "Time for the dreaded Monday morning laundry routine," she thought, as she gathered up her dirty clothes and rounded up a handful of quarters. As she sorted out her coloreds and whites, she saw spotting on her underwear from the day before. "Bummer, I thought that had disappeared," she puzzled. Heather stopped loading the clothes and went to the bathroom to investigate. Sure enough, the spotting was back again today. Heather had finished her period over a week ago, so she didn't think it could be from that.

Heather thought, "I guess I didn't notice my underwear last night, since I got changed in the dark." Heather and Scott were becoming regular night owls, so Heather had started getting ready for bed with the light off so she wouldn't wake her roommate when she came in from a late date. Heather's thoughts drifted back to last night. "I can't believe how we love all the same things—Asian food, mountain biking, and watching old movies. It's almost too good to be true." She quickly knocked on wood, warding off any jinx her thoughts may have triggered. "Okay, Heather, focus," she sternly told herself and grabbed the campus phone book to find the number for the health center.

Just a few hours later, Heather was on an exam table, nervously sitting half naked with a sheet draped over her legs. The nurse, Maureen, was setting out scary-looking equipment on a nearby tray table. "What's that?" Heather asked apprehensively.

"This is a pelvic speculum, and this smaller one is an anoscope," Maureen replied matter-of-factly. "Haven't you had a pelvic exam before?" she asked.

"No, I most certainly have not," exclaimed Heather. "Does the doctor have to put that thing inside me? It looks huge."

"Really, it's not that bad," reassured Maureen, "you'll feel some pressure, but not pain."

"But I'm a virgin," protested Heather. "I mean, I use tampons, but that is way bigger than one of those."

"Don't worry, Dr. Jones is really gentle. I'll be sure to tell him that this will be your first pelvic exam. If you just have hemorrhoids, he might be able to see that without even using any of this. Just relax, and he and I will be back in the room in a minute."

Heather swallowed hard as Maureen whisked out of the room and closed the door. She shifted back and forth on the table, way too nervous to just "relax" as the nurse had suggested. Her eyes were drawn to the tray table, focusing on the two instruments and numerous swabs that had been set out. "All this for a little spotting," thought Heather. "Maybe I overreacted, and I really don't need any of this." She was seriously thinking about getting dressed and leaving, when Maureen and the doctor came in.

Dr. Jones had dark, thick hair and a mustache. He was short and stocky, with a muscular chest and arms. His light blue button-down shirt was neatly pressed, matching his starched white coat. "Hi, I'm Dr. Jones," he greeted Heather, extending his hand. "So I understand that you've noticed some spotting on your underwear, is that right?"

"Yes, just a couple of times," answered Heather.

"When did you first notice it?"

"About a month ago, on a Friday night. At first I thought I was going to start my period, but then by the next day, the spotting was gone," said Heather. "I didn't notice any again until today."

"And now you think it's coming from your rectum?" inquired Dr. Jones.

"I think so. Do people my age get hemorrhoids?"

"Actually, hemorrhoids are fairly common in college students, because their diet is often pretty low in fiber. Are you a burger and pizza girl, or do you try to maintain a healthy diet?" asked Dr. Jones.

"To be honest, I think I eat far better than the average college student," Heather bragged. "I grew up always making sure to eat plenty of fruits and vegetables, so I have a banana with breakfast most days, and I always snack on apples and grapes. My friends actually tease me because I also love those high-fiber snack bars."

"Have you had any diarrhea or constipation lately?" he asked.

"Not that I've noticed," she replied.

Dr. Jones made some notes in her chart, and then he looked up. "I see that you have regular periods, and that you have not been sexually active yet. Is that correct?"

Heather blushed. "That's right."

"Okay, then. Let me have you lie back so we can make sure you don't have any extra lumps or bumps anywhere, and we'll see what seems to be causing this spotting."

Heather began to lie back on the table as Maureen stepped over and pulled out stirrups from the end of the table. "Oh, speaking of bumps, last month I thought I felt some small ones around my bottom when I saw that spotting, but I couldn't see anything with a mirror."

Dr. Jones and Maureen exchanged a look, which didn't escape notice by Heather.

Casually, Dr. Jones continued his questions. "What kind of bumps? Could you see or feel how big they were?"

"They were small, maybe pea-sized. Does that sound like a hemorrhoid?" she asked hopefully. She felt sweat break out on her palms.

"Just go ahead and lie back, and we'll take a look," he said.

Heather followed his directions, trying to keep her knees apart as Maureen gently directed her. She watched Dr. Jones put on his gloves and begin to examine her.

Almost immediately, he reported, "Okay, I see the problem here. I need to use this small scope to look inside, though. Just try and relax, and I'll be done in a minute."

Before she knew it, Heather felt the instrument enter her rectum. She thought she might die from embarrassment or fear, but the procedure was done fairly quickly. Or so she thought.

"Okay, now I need to do the pelvic exam," Dr. Jones revealed.

"What?" Heather sat halfway up, rising up on her elbows, but with her feet still in the stirrups. "Do you remember that I haven't had sex yet?" she protested.

"Look, Heather, here's the deal. You've got anal warts, which is a sexually transmitted disease. I need to look in your vagina to make sure that you don't have any warts inside," Dr. Jones said.

Heather was incredulous. She thought to herself, "Anal warts? How disgusting can you get? And how in the heck did I get them without having sex?" But she didn't say anything, simply fell back and endured the pelvic exam.

"Okay, you can sit up now. We did a Pap smear, which tests for the wart virus on your cervix, and checked you for other STDs. The only warts that I saw in the exam were the few near your anus, and they aren't bleeding right now. I assume that's what's causing your spotting," the doctor said.

"Are you sure it's warts?" Heather asked.

"Yes, Heather. We see these pretty frequently. Typically, it's from anal sex. Do you think that might be how you got yours?" he asked gently.

Tears filled Heather's eyes. "I swear," she sobbed. "It was one time, and it wasn't my idea. At the end of the summer, my old high school boyfriend and I were together for the last time before he left to go back to college." The doctor looked uncomfortable, but Maureen smiled and touched Heather's knee sympathetically. Heather rushed through the rest of her explanation. "He brought over this really expensive bottle of wine, and we drank the whole thing. I don't even drink usually, so I was pretty drunk, and when we fooled around, things got out of control. He kept trying to put it in my rear, telling me I'd still be a virgin. I stopped him, though. I didn't let him actually do it." Heather broke down.

"I'm sorry," said Dr. Jones, "but if you'd like me to start treating the warts today, I'll need you to lie back down. It's going to sting a bit. Maureen, can you grab the liquid nitrogen from the cabinet?"

"*Start* treating them? How long does it take?" Heather asked.

"I don't know yet how many times you'll need. We'll have to see you back in two weeks, and likely repeat the treatment. Usually, it takes several visits to get rid of a crop of these warts. Luckily, I didn't see any inside your rectum or your vagina. That would have been a much bigger deal. We send those to the specialists to treat."

"What are you going to use on me today?" Heather asked. Dr. Jones held up the bottle Maureen had just handed him and showed it to Heather. "I prefer treating warts like yours with liquid nitrogen. TCA, which is an acid, can also be used, but it can be a little tough on the anal area. There is another milder medicine that patients can use at home, but I find it is not as successful. Besides, where your warts are, they're pretty hard for you to see, so honestly, I think you'll do much better if we just treat you here."

"As long as you get rid of them, I'm with you," sighed Heather, lying back once again and finding the stirrups with her feet.

Dr. Jones began to apply the liquid nitrogen, and Heather realized she was biting her lip to keep from crying. Sharp burning pain made it nearly impossible to keep her legs open as the doctor treated the warts. "How many are there?" Heather managed to squeak out between applications.

"Looks like there are just four," replied Dr. Jones. "Okay, I'm finished." He walked around the side of the exam table so he could look directly at Heather. "Please schedule an appointment for two weeks from now, and we'll repeat this treatment again. These warts should completely disappear within two to three months."

"Months?"

"Yes, months. But, Heather, just because these warts disappear, it doesn't mean the virus is gone," he finished. "Also, about twenty-five percent of people with newly diagnosed anal warts have a recurrence within the first three months after treatment."

Heather rose up on her elbows again, challenging "What? I thought you said this treatment would make them go away."

"All warts are caused by a virus, Heather, and we don't yet have a cure for the virus. Maureen will get you a handout that explains all this. The virus is called HPV, which stands for the human papilloma virus. There are lots of different strains of HPV. Types six and eleven cause the vast majority of genital warts, roughly ninety percent, but they don't seem to cause cancer. It is possible, though less likely, for genital or anal warts to be caused by other strains of HPV that can cause vulvar, anal, or penile cancer. Types sixteen and eighteen have the strongest link to cervical cancer but rarely cause visible warts like you have."

Heather lay back down and closed her eyes, confused and speechless. Dr. Jones continued, "Also, I recommend that you get the new vaccine Gardasil today. I'm hoping your Pap smear doesn't show any type of HPV infection, but we know you have at least one type of HPV causing your warts. Gardasil works against all four HPV types that I mentioned—types six and eleven that cause genital warts, and types sixteen and eighteen, which cause seventy percent of all cervical cancers. The vaccine is a series of three injections that you receive over six months. It's believed that the majority of sexually active adults harbor the HPV infection, although most don't know it because they don't have symptoms. In fact, the Centers for Disease Control say that more than twenty million Americans at any given time have active HPV, and roughly seventy-five percent of Americans aged fifteen to forty-nine years old have been infected at some point. Obviously, this makes HPV by far the most common STD in the United States. Chances are that you don't yet have the types of HPV that cause cervical cancer, and the vaccine would help you avoid getting it."

"So you're telling me that I'm stuck with this virus forever, even if we make the warts go away, and even if I get the vaccine. Is that right?" Heather asked.

"Yes. However, as long as we treat outbreaks and screen you regularly, my hope is that it won't bother you that much," replied Dr. Jones. "When you decide to be sexually active in the future, you need to let your partner know that you have the virus. We think condoms reduce the risk for HPV-related diseases, meaning warts and cancer. Condoms are not by any means foolproof, though, because the virus can be present on areas that condoms don't cover, like the scrotum or anus in guys, or the vulva or anus in girls. Does that make sense?"

Heather nodded in agreement, trying to process everything the doctor had said and doing her best to ignore the searing pain in her bottom.

"Okay, then, I'll see you in a couple weeks," Dr. Jones said as he left the room.

Maureen put away her supplies and turned back to Heather, peeking under her drape to check the warts. "Alright, honey, you can get up now. I put a two-pack of ibuprofen on the counter for you to help with the discomfort, right next to the HPV handout. I'll give you a few minutes to get dressed, then I'll come back with your first dose of Gardasil, assuming you want to get it."

"Absolutely," said Heather. "I still can't believe I've got *any* kind of wart virus. If that shot will keep me from getting other ones, I'm all for it." Heather shook her head incredulously. "Frankly, it sounds to me that if I would have gotten the vaccine a few years ago, I wouldn't be sitting here right now, right?"

"Don't beat yourself up about it, Heather," reassured Maureen. "Gardasil was only approved by the FDA in June 2006, so it's not surprising you haven't had it yet."

Heather got dressed, received her vaccine, and scheduled her follow-up appointment. She carefully walked across campus, trying not to aggravate her sores, oblivious to the sunshine and crisp weather. "Anal warts. I have anal warts. Oh my gosh, how did I let this happen?" The thoughts were stuck in her head, playing over and over with every painful step toward her dorm. "Does Darren even know he has HPV? He's always so lucky, I'll bet he never even had a wart. Warts. Anal warts," and she was back in the painful loop again. As Heather opened the door to her dorm, her cell phone chirped, alerting Heather of a new text. "Great Day. Let's bike. Call me, S."

Tears overflowing once again, Heather could only think sarcastically, "Oh yeah, great day. Sure, sitting on a bike seat with my rear end on fire sounds absolutely wonderful right now." But she knew her real anger wasn't directed at Scott. The reality of her disease was sinking in. What would she tell Scott? Would she tell him? What would she think if Scott told her that he had anal warts? It was just too much to absorb right now. Heather typed back, "Sorry, today's packed. Rain check? J."

"One step at a time," she thought. "I'll figure it out. Me and the twenty million other Americans."

facts

Human Papilloma Virus (HPV) Fact Sheet

What is it?

- The human papilloma virus (HPV) is a group of over one hundred viral subtypes, more than 30 of which are transmitted sexually.

- Types 16 and 18 cause 70% of cervical cancers.

- Types 6 and 11 cause 90% of genital warts.

- Other types cause "common" warts on hands or feet.

How common is it?

- The CDC estimates that 20 million people, 15% of the population, are actively infected at any given time with sexually transmitted HPV in the United States, although many more people do not know they are infected.

- 6.2 million Americans are newly infected each year.

- HPV is thought to be the most common sexually transmitted infection in the United States.

- Over one million people have visible genital warts at any given time in the United States.

How do you get it?

- Through skin-to-skin contact with an infected partner, with the thin skin of the genitals being most easily infected. (HPV does not live in blood, semen, or vaginal secretions.)

- Through oral, vaginal, or anal sex.

- Less commonly, HPV genital wart types can be passed to a baby during vaginal childbirth, causing serious problems with warts in the infant's larynx, eyes, or genitals.

Where on your body do you get it?

- In women, genital warts can occur on the labia, vagina, cervix, anywhere in the anal or genital area, and on the abdomen or thighs.

- In men, genital warts can occur in the urethral opening, on the penis, scrotum, or anus, and on the abdomen or thighs.

How do I know if I have it?

- Most people are asymptomatic and may only be diagnosed on a routine checkup.

- Pap smears may detect all types of HPV.

- A small percentage of people infected with HPV grow genital warts, which are usually painless.

- Warts in the opening of the urethra can cause blood in the urine.

- Warts can itch or bleed, though most do not.

- Coating the genitals with vinegar can make warts turn white, making them easier to see; however, other benign skin conditions may also turn white.

What does it look like?

- Normal anatomy or flesh-colored flat or raised wrinkled bumps, single or in groups.

What does it feel like?

- Most people are unaware that they have HPV.

- 20% of people with genital warts experience itching.

How long does it last?

- It is believed that, once infected with a type of HPV, you will have that type for the rest of your life.

- 20% of genital warts resolve without treatment (meaning the visible warts disappear, but the infection remains).

- 25% of genital warts recur in the first three months after treatment.

Can it be cured?

- No. Treatments can remove visible warts, but recurrence is common, and infectivity is permanent.

- Infectivity is thought to be greater when there are untreated, visible warts.

Can you be re-infected?

- Not with the same strain of HPV.

- Rarely, people autoinoculate themselves, meaning they transmit HPV from the genitals to another location on their own body.

What is the treatment?

- Multiple treatments exist, and type of treatment depends on location, number, and size of warts, as well as physician and patient preference.

Treatments performed by providers:
- Cryotherapy: freezing with liquid nitrogen; treatments repeated every one to two weeks until warts have resolved.
- TCA or BCA: acids that chemically burn the warts; dries to a white crust; can be repeated every one to two weeks until warts are resolved.
- Podophyllin: applied to wart and often washed off 1 to 4 hours later; not indicated for pregnant women.
- Laser: usually for extensive warts, intraurethral warts, or those resistant to other therapy.
- Surgery: treatment is usually complete in one visit; higher risk of scarring.

Treatments applied by patients (should be discussed with physician first):

- Podoflox: applied with swab twice daily for 3 days, then 4 days without treatment; cycle may be repeated up to 4 cycles. Ideally, physician should perform first application to confirm warts and safety of this method.
- Imiquod: applied at bedtime 3 nights per week for up to 16 weeks; washed off 6 to 10 hours later.

How about alternative therapies?

- Interferon injections directly into wart lesions are not recommended as a primary treatment due to high side effects and necessity of multiple treatments.

- No herbal or home remedies are proven to eliminate HPV.

- Swabbing of the genital area with vinegar may help patients and partners identify new warts.

Are there long-term consequences of HPV?

- Types 16 and 18 cause 70% of cervical cancer.

- Types 16, 18, 31, 33, and 35 are considered the high-risk types of HPV because of their link with cervical, vaginal, anal, and other squamous cell cancers, and they can all be occasionally found in genital warts, although 90% of genital warts are caused by types 6 and 11, which are not precancerous.

When are you contagious?

- Any time you are infected with HPV, regardless of symptoms.

- Even while using a condom. Latex male condoms can reduce but not eliminate transmission of HPV, since HPV is present on genital surfaces not covered with a condom.

How do I avoid getting HPV?

- Completely abstaining from oral, vaginal, and anal sex, as well as direct skin-to-skin genital contact, is the only way to be 100% sure to avoid contracting HPV.

- Gardasil vaccine offers protection against HPV types 6 and 11, which cause 90% of genital warts, and types 16 and 18, which cause 70% of cervical cancers.

- Condoms are thought to only moderately decrease transmission of HPV.

If I have HPV, how do I avoid giving it to my partner?

- If your partner is female, she should be immunized with the Gardasil vaccine to protect her from getting HPV types 6, 11, 16, and 18. (Gardasil is not offered to males at this time.)

- Condom use is recommended, but effectiveness in preventing transmission of HPV is questionable.

- Direct skin-to-skin contact involving the genital area of an infected person can transmit HPV, so abstain from "dry humping" (genital contact without vaginal or anal penetration) as well as intercourse.

Does HPV transmission occur in homosexual partners?

- HPV is transmitted through skin-to-skin contact with an infected partner, regardless of gender.

- HPV transmission does occur in women who have sex with women, although documentation is limited (due to many studies including women who have bisexual as well as homosexual contacts).

- HPV can be contracted through receiving anal intercourse.

Frequently Asked Questions

➤ How common is HPV?
There are more than 20 million Americans with this virus.

➤ Will my genital warts turn into cancer?
Although the risk is not zero, it's very unlikely.

➤ If I just developed warts, did my current partner cheat on me?
No, most likely not. The HPV virus can be dormant for weeks, months, years, or even a lifetime. It is not known what triggers an outbreak of warts, although stress and immune status are thought to play a role.

Your partner may be one of the many Americans with silent, and therefore, undiagnosed HPV.

➤ To catch HPV, do you have to have sex with multiple partners?
No. Although your risk of any STD increases with the number of partners you have had, HPV is so common that you can easily contract it from even your first partner (unless neither of you has had any prior genital contact).

➤ If I get the Gardasil vaccine, will I still need to use condoms?
Yes. Gardasil only works against HPV. The injection offers no protection from any other sexually transmitted disease.

➤ Can my male partner be tested for HPV?
There are no tests currently available to screen men for HPV.

Additional Information

American College of Obstetricians and Gynecologists
P. O. Box 96920
409 12th Street, SW
Washington, DC 20090-6920
202-863-2518
www.acog.org/departments/dept_notice.cfm?recno=7&bulletin
=3097

American Social Health Association
P. O. Box 13827
Research Triangle Park, NC 27709
1-800-227-8922
www.ashastd.org/hpv/hpv_overview.cfm

CDC-INFO
Centers for Disease Control and Prevention
1600 Clifton Road
Atlanta, GA 30333
1-800-CDC-INFO (1-800-232-4636), 1-888-232-6348 TTY
www.cdc.gov/std/hpv/default.htm

Centers for Disease Control and Prevention
HPV Vaccine—Questions and Answers
www.cdc.gov/vaccines/vpd-vac/hpv/vac-faqs.htm

MedlinePlus
National Library of Medicine
8600 Rockville Pike
Bethesda, MD 20894
1-888-FIND-NLM (1-888-346-3656), or 301-594-5983
www.nlm.nih.gov/medlineplus/hpv.html

National Cancer Institute
Public Inquiries Office
6116 Executive Boulevard, Room 3036A
Bethesda, MD 20892-8322
1-800-4-CANCER (1-800-422-6237)
www.cancer.gov/cancertopics/factsheet/Risk/HPV

CERVICAL CANCER

5: Lisa

LISA HAD BEEN SITTING in the waiting room of the gynecologist for over an hour. As a grade-school art teacher, it was extremely difficult to get time off to go to the doctor, and if she didn't get done soon, she was afraid she wouldn't make it back to teach the afternoon classes. The nurse had come out a while ago to tell everyone that Dr. Butler had been called away to an emergency delivery, asking if anyone wanted to reschedule. Lisa had been somewhat amazed that most ladies declined and went right back to reading various parenting magazines. One lady with a tiny baby and another with an active toddler went up to the check-in area and apparently rescheduled and left.

Lisa looked around at the obviously pregnant ladies and wondered how soon it would be her turn to have a child. Lisa was twenty-four years old and had been married just over three years. Her husband, Jack, was a civil engineer. He was a compulsively organized, predictable kind of guy. Lisa was much more of a free spirit. They were the ultimate "opposites attract" couple, but their extremes complemented one another beautifully.

Jack did all the finances, from paying bills to investments. Lisa was in charge of their social life, cooking, and home décor. She loved to host elaborately themed wine tastings or holiday parties. They both loved kids and talked about raising three or four of their own. Lisa wasn't desperate to start trying to conceive, but as more of her friends had babies, she was happy that she and Jack had decided to stop using birth control and let nature take its course this year.

At Jack's insistence, Lisa had gone to see her family physician to get a full physical and "clearance," as he put it, that she was in optimal health and ready to conceive. Lisa had laughed at his concern, telling him that nothing could be wrong with her since she had become a vegetarian and avid yoga practitioner a couple of years ago. Indeed, everything turned out great, except for Lisa's Pap smear.

The nurse had told Lisa that the Pap smear is a screening test for cervical cancer. (Lisa had explained to Jack that the cervix is the opening to the "womb" where the baby grows.) Apparently, Lisa had some abnormal cells that the doctor was worried about. Lisa recalled that she had a couple of Pap smears during college that were "mildly abnormal," but no one ever said she needed anything other than a repeat Pap test. Now her doctor was concerned enough to refer her to the gynecologist for further testing, which is why Lisa had scheduled this appointment.

Apparently, she was in for a "pretty uncomfortable" experience that included "biopsies" of her cervix. She had taken a bunch of ibuprofen prior to this appointment, as the office had instructed when she scheduled it. Lisa didn't want to reschedule an appointment that she had been somewhat dreading and had rearranged her schedule for.

Finally, about an hour and a half later than her scheduled appointment time, she was brought back into an exam room. The medical assistant, Shelly, took all her vital signs and gave her a patient gown. Shelly clearly had copies of Lisa's Pap smear report, and she reviewed with her the game plan for the day. She also needed to review Lisa's gynecological history.

"So, how old were you when your periods started?" Shelly inquired.

"Gosh, I don't know. I think seventh grade—what is that, like twelve years old?" Lisa responded.

"Sounds right," Shelly agreed. "And are your periods regular?"

"Well, yes, but I've been on the pill for a lot of years," said Lisa.
Shelly continued, "Any spotting or bleeding between periods?"

"No, not really," Lisa replied.

"Have you ever been pregnant?" asked Shelly.

"No, but we're planning to start trying this year."

"Great. Maybe you'll be back soon as an obstetrical patient," Shelly added enthusiastically. "Okay, back to my form. Are you now, or have you ever been, a smoker?"

"Oh, in college I used to smoke socially, but I haven't had a cigarette in years now," replied Lisa.

"Good for you," approved Shelly. "How many total sexual partners have you had? One to five, six to ten, or greater than ten?"

Lisa actually blushed at this question. She had always been very comfortable with her sexuality, but counting up her encounters seemed crass. She thought about it for a moment, then opted to round down a touch and said, "in the six range."

"And any history of sexually transmitted diseases?" Shelly asked.

Lisa was more prepared for this question. "Well, yes, in college I was treated for chlamydia once."

"Anything else?"

"No, not that I can think of," Lisa replied.

"What about the human papilloma virus?" Shelly asked.

"The what?" asked Lisa.

"The wart virus. Actually, that's what you've got now, but I was trying to find out if this was the first time it had showed up on your Pap smear," Shelly said, apologetically.

"Oh," said Lisa. "Actually, they just told me my Pap smear was abnormal, but I didn't realize it was from a wart virus. That's weird, because I don't think I have any warts."

Shelly reassured Lisa that the majority of the patients they saw with abnormal changes from this virus did not have any associated warts. "The problem is that you tested positive for the types of this virus, which we call HPV, that are high risk for causing cervical cancer. That's why we brought you here to take a look and do a few biopsies to see how best to treat you," explained Shelly.

"Wait, are you saying I could have cancer? Or that I have a wart virus? I'm confused," said Lisa.

Shelly elaborated, "All we know right now is that you have this virus, HPV. And, yes, HPV can cause cancer. However, we'll need the results from the biopsies that the doctor will take today to tell us exactly how much, if any, precancerous change you actually have."

"Could it be cancer already?" worried Lisa.

"It's very unlikely in your case, because your Pap smear was only mildly abnormal," answered Shelly.

Lisa nodded, but now her heart was racing. She had known that a Pap smear was a test for cervical cancer, but everyone had seemed so calm about her abnormal test, it hadn't really clicked with her that there could be a serious problem. "But we'll know for sure once the doctor looks at the biopsies? Will that be today?"

"Yes, that should tell us everything we need to know. It's a pathologist who looks at the biopsies, but it takes a few days to get the results. We'll certainly call you as soon as we hear."

"A few days to worry about whether or not I've got cancer. Great," thought Lisa. She decided she'd better focus on the moment, and what to expect from the upcoming procedure.

"Now I'm pretty nervous. Do you knock me out or something? I'm kind of wimpy about pain."

Shelly smiled, "Oh, no. It's like a regular Pap smear, but with a pain that feels like a hard menstrual cramp for most people. Did you take some ibuprofen this morning?"

"Yes."

"Then really, that's all you'll need. Dr. Butler ought to be here pretty soon, and she'll answer any more questions you might have."

Shelly then went over the consent form for colposcopy and biopsies and handed it to Lisa to sign. "You're her first patient when she gets back," said Shelly, "so she should be here any minute."

"Don't worry, I've waited this long, so I'm not going anywhere," Lisa replied.

Dr. Butler popped in the door a few minutes later, with Shelly following in behind her. "Hi, I'm Dr. Butler," she said. "Sorry I'm running so far behind, but I was called out for a delivery. Anyway, I'm here now, so let's get started. I'm sure you're anxious to get this over with."

"Definitely," replied Lisa.

"I see you had an abnormal Pap smear, and we found cells that can cause cervical cancer, so you're here for further treatment. Did Shelly go over everything with you?"

"Pretty much," Lisa shrugged tensely.

"Good. Go ahead and lie back and scoot down," said the doctor.

Lisa did as the doctor instructed, and the next five minutes or so passed in a blur as Lisa used her meditation skills to try to relax to minimize the discomfort. Lisa certainly thought it hurt way more than a menstrual cramp, but she didn't say anything.

"Okay, we're finished. It will take a few days until we get the results back from the pathologist, and Shelly will call you with your results. Meanwhile, let me give you my speech about HPV, okay?"

Lisa was sitting up now, relieved the procedure was over but uncomfortable, and ready to focus on what the doctor was telling her. "Fire away," she said.

"Okay, here goes. HPV, the human papilloma virus, is extremely common. They estimate that an American's lifetime risk of acquiring it is nearly seventy-five percent. Risk factors for getting it are multiple sexual partners or sex with one high-risk partner, smoking, and a history of having other STDs. There is debate about whether oral contraceptive pills increase or decrease the risk. There are many types of HPV, but only a few are responsible for causing cervical cancer. Another couple of types cause most of warts—both genital and in other locations like the hands or legs. You are here because your Pap smear and a DNA test showed that you have the type of HPV that is high risk for causing cancer, so we needed to actually get some tissue samples to make sure that you don't already have cancerous changes."

"Did it look like cancer to you?" interjected Lisa.

"To the naked eye, it looks normal. The whole point, though, is to find any precancerous or even cancerous cells as early as possible, before it gets to the point where it would be visible on a pelvic exam. If we find any of those cells on your biopsies, then we will need to do another procedure to get rid of those cells and try to prevent any progression towards cancer. Are you with me so far?" she asked.

"Yes," said Lisa. "So I definitely have this wart virus, specifically, the kind that wants to cause cancer, not warts, but we don't know yet if it has caused any cancer changes?"

"Exactly," said Dr. Butler.

"And will this affect me getting pregnant?" asked Lisa.

"Not the procedure you've just finished. It would depend what extra procedures you might need if the biopsies show any cancerous changes," said Dr. Butler.

"So there's no antibiotic to fix this, just surgeries?" asked Lisa.

"Not yet. However, you've probably seen ads for the new HPV vaccine, Gardasil, that recently came out on the market. We're really optimistic that it will help to virtually eliminate cervical cancer for our next generation of women. This vaccine will protect against HPV types 16 and 18, which cause seventy percent of cervical cancer. As a bonus, it also protects against types 6 and 11, which make up ninety percent of genital warts. Prevention will be our best tool to fight cervical cancer because, unfortunately, there are not any antiviral medicines that work yet," admitted the doctor.

"And what about my husband? Does he need to be tested or treated?" Lisa wondered.

"The only way we're aware that a man has HPV is when he develops genital warts. If you remember what I said earlier, the strain that we know you have can cause cancer, but is highly unlikely to cause warts. So, while we know your husband has been exposed and is most likely infected, we don't yet have any way to detect or treat this strain of virus in him."

"So basically, we just wait to see my results and hope I don't need any further treatment?" said Lisa.

"Well, yes. We will call you next week and let you know," said Dr. Butler.

"And if it is cancerous? Can you tell me what to expect then?" said Lisa.

"It would depend on the pathology report. Often, we can treat patients with a quick procedure here in the office, using chemicals or liquid nitrogen to destroy the tissue. We also have surgical options, using lasers or loops to remove the tissue. Of course, you would be sedated for those procedures," replied Dr. Butler.

"Are all cervical cancers caused by this HPV?" asked Lisa.

"We think so. It's amazing to think that an STD causes cancer, isn't it?" answered the doctor.

"Wait—you consider this an STD even when there are no warts?" Lisa asked doubtfully.

"Definitely. STD means that you caught this through sex, and that is the only way this disease is transmitted."

Lisa let that sink in for a moment and then asked, "So, how often does the virus actually cause cancer? Does anyone ever die of cervical cancer any more?"

"Sadly, yes. Cervical cancer is the second most common cancer in women worldwide, but it doesn't get as much press as breast cancer, even though cervical cancer is preventable. In 2001, there were 12,900 cases of cervical cancer in the United States, with nearly 5,000 deaths from it that year," said Dr. Butler. We've only had one patient in our practice die from it, but that was one too many. I'm not telling you this to scare you, but to emphasize the seriousness of the effects of HPV. With our improving detection of early cellular changes and ability to detect the high-risk HPV strains, we are able to cure the vast majority of the cancers that we find."

Well, that certainly put a stronger slant on the whole thing. Lisa made a mental note to thank her diligent husband for pushing her to get that physical. "Well, you've certainly got my attention. I truly had no idea this could be that serious. I guess I'll talk to you ladies next week, then," she said, and thanked both the doctor and her medical assistant. Lisa got dressed and checked out.

As she walked through the waiting room, she looked at the pregnant ladies with new appreciation. Lisa realized that things she had taken for granted even an hour ago now meant more to her. She looked forward to the time when, rather than dreading a procedure to treat the wart virus, she would be sitting in this room excited to hear her baby's heartbeat. Lisa hoped and prayed she hadn't lost that chance already.

facts

Cervical Cancer Fact Sheet

What is it?

- Cervical cancer is a disease of uncontrolled growth of abnormal cells of the cervix, which is the lower part, or opening, of the uterus.

- Human papilloma virus types 16 and 18 cause 70% of cervical cancers.

- HPV types 16, 18, 31, 33, and 35 are considered the high-risk HPV types because of their link with cervical, vaginal, anal, and other squamous cell cancers.

- 5 to 30% of infections will include more than one type of HPV.

How common is it?

- The National Cancer Institute estimates that 11,070 women in the United States will be diagnosed with invasive cervical cancer in 2008.

- There will be roughly 3,870 deaths in the United States from cervical cancer in 2008.

- Keep in mind that, although the majority (50-75%) of sexually active adults in the United States will at some point acquire HPV, only a small percentage will develop cervical cancer.

- 6 out of 10 women who developed cervical cancer in 2004 had not had a Pap test in more than 5 years, if ever.

How do you get it?

- Skin-to-skin contact or intercourse with an infected partner carrying the human papilloma virus can transmit HPV, which causes cervical cancer.

Where on your body do you get it?

- Cervical cancer starts on the cervix but can extend to include the vaginal wall, uterus, rectum, bladder, lymph nodes, lungs, liver, or other sites.

How do I know if I have it?

- Early on, most are asymptomatic and may only be diagnosed during a routine checkup.

- Pap smears detect the types of HPV that cause cervical cancer.

- Not all abnormal Pap smears are precancerous or cancerous;

your healthcare professional can explain what your abnormal Pap smear means.

What does it look like?

- Normal anatomy, or red, inflamed cervix. A growth may be visible at late stages.

What does it feel like?

- Most people are unaware they have cervical cancer because at early stages, there are usually no symptoms.

- In more advanced disease, the woman may notice abnormal vaginal bleeding, including bleeding or spotting between periods, after intercourse, or after menopause and/or menstrual periods that are longer or heavier than normal.

- Increased vaginal discharge, pelvic pain, and dysparunia (pain with intercourse) can be present in advanced disease.

- Bleeding after intercourse—1 in 220 women with this symptom have invasive cervical cancer.

What is a Pap smear or Pap test?

- A Pap smear is a test for cervical cancer. A medical professional inserts an instrument into the vagina so they can see the cervix and then uses a brush or cotton-tipped applicator to collect cells from the cervix. This specimen is sent to a cytology lab, where a cytotechnologist looks at the cells under a microscope. If any abnormalities are detected, the smear is routed to a pathologist for further evaluation.

Who needs a Pap test?

- Any woman who has had sexual intercourse and has not had a hysterectomy should have a Pap test for cervical cancer.

- Women over 65 who have never had an abnormal Pap test and women who have had a hysterectomy that includes removal of the cervix do not need a Pap test.

How do I prepare for the Pap test?

- Do not have sex, douche, use tampons, or use any vaginal cream, gel, or foam (including spermicides) for two days prior to your Pap test.

- Schedule your Pap test for a time when you should not be having your period.

Can it be cured?

- Yes. Many cervical cancers are caught early and can be cured with treatment.

Can you be re-infected?

- Cancer can recur.

What are the basic stages of cervical cancer?

- Stage 0: The cancer is found only in the top layer of cells in the tissue that lines the cervix. Stage 0 is also called carcinoma in situ.

- Stage I: The cancer has invaded the cervix beneath the top layer of cells. It is found only in the cervix.

- Stage II: The cancer extends beyond the cervix into nearby tissues. It extends to the upper part of the vagina. The cancer does not invade the lower third of the vagina or the pelvic wall (the lining of the part of the body between the hips).

- Stage III: The cancer extends to the lower part of the vagina. It also may have spread to the pelvic wall and nearby lymph nodes.

- Stage IV: The cancer has spread to the bladder, rectum, or other parts of the body.

What is the treatment?

- Multiple treatments exist, and type of treatment depends on staging of the disease. Thanks to Pap tests, most cervical cancers are discovered at stage 0 or stage 1 and therefore are easily treated. Treatments include:

  - Surgery: In stage 0 (very early cancer), surgical treatment can be performed that leaves the uterus intact, allowing the possibility of future childbearing. More advanced stages may require removal of the uterus, fallopian tubes, and ovaries.
  - Chemotherapy.
  - Radiation.
  - Combination of any of the above methods.

How about alternative therapies?

- No herbal or home remedies are proven to eliminate cervical cancer.

Are there long-term consequences?

- Infertility, if there is scarring from the treatment; more common at stage I and beyond.

- Death, an estimated 3,870 women die from cervical cancer each year in the United States.

When are you contagious?

- Any time you are infected with HPV, regardless of symptoms, you are contagious. However, you can only transmit the virus, not cervical cancer itself.

- Latex male condoms can reduce but not eliminate transmission of HPV, as HPV is present on genital surfaces not covered with a condom.

How can I avoid getting cervical cancer?

- Abstinence or monogamy with a partner who has had no prior sexual partners will prevent getting HPV, which causes cervical cancer.

- Gardasil vaccine prevents infection with HPV types 16 and 18, which cause 70% of cervical cancers.

Frequently Asked Questions

➤ How many abnormal Pap tests turn out to be invasive cancer?
Out of 50 million Pap tests annually, roughly 2 million are abnormal, and only 11,000 are invasive cancers.

➤ Does smoking cause cervical cancer?
The human papilloma virus causes cervical cancer, but women with HPV who smoke have a higher incidence of cervical cancer than those with HPV who do not smoke.

➤ Will my genital warts turn into cancer?
Although the risk is not zero, it's very unlikely. Different strains

of HPV cause warts than those that typically cause cancer.

➤ **If I have cervical cancer, does that count as an STD?**
Yes. We now know that cervical cancers are caused by the human papilloma virus (HPV), although risk factors like smoking, weakened immune system, age over 40, and lack of regular Pap tests do contribute.

➤ **To catch HPV, do you have to have sex with multiple partners?**
No. Although your risk of any STD increases with the number of partners you have had, HPV is so widespread that you can easily contract it even from your first partner (unless you both have had no prior genital contact).

➤ **If I get the Gardasil vaccine, can I still get cervical cancer?**
Yes. Gardasil protects against the types of HPV that cause 70% of cervical cancers, so there is still the possibility of contracting the types of HPV that cause the other 30% of cervical cancers.

➤ **If I get the Gardasil vaccine, do I need to use condoms?**
Yes. Gardasil protects against four types of HPV but no other STDs.

Additional Information

American College of Obstetricians and Gynecologists
P. O. Box 96920
409 12th Street, SW
Washington, DC 20090-6920
202-863-2518
www.acog.org/publications/patient_education/bp163.cfm

American Social Health Association
P. O. Box 13827
Research Triangle Park, NC 27709
1-800-227-8922
www.ashastd.org/hpv/hpv_learn_women.cfm

CDC-INFO
Centers for Disease Control and Prevention
1600 Clifton Road
Atlanta, GA 30333
1-800-CDC-INFO (1-800-232-4636), 1-888-232-6348 TTY
www.cdc.gov/cancer/cervical/

Centers for Disease Control and Prevention
HPV Vaccine Questions and Answers
www.cdc.gov/vaccines/vpd-vac/hpv/vac-faqs.htm

MedlinePlus
National Library of Medicine
8600 Rockville Pike
Bethesda, MD 20894
1-888-FIND-NLM (1-888-346-3656), or 301-594-5983
www.nlm.nih.gov/medlineplus/cervicalcancer.html

National Cancer Institute
Public Inquiries Office
6116 Executive Boulevard, Room 3036A
Bethesda, MD 20892-8322
1-800-4-CANCER (1-800-422-6237)
www.cancer.gov/cancertopics/types/cervical

CHLAMYDIA

6: Tony

TONY WINCED AS HE finished urinating. "Ouch, that hurt," he thought. "I guess I must have had too much to drink." Over the weekend, he had downed at least a twelve-pack of beer during an all-day fraternity party, not to mention the Seagram's that he and his friends had snuck into the game to spice up their Cokes. Basketball season was always awesome, but the hangovers after the games weren't so much fun. Last weekend had been especially crazy, with the road trip to meet his college's cross-state rivals.

To top it all off, Tony had hooked up with his ex-girlfriend, Tami, when she showed up at the party. There had been one pretty embarrassing moment, however, when they had sex after the game. He couldn't believe that he had drank enough to make it difficult to keep an erection. He'd heard guys joke about "whiskey dick" but hadn't believed it happened to nineteen-year-olds. Thank goodness Tami was cool with him taking off the condom so he could "feel" more. After that, he had no problems.

He and Tami had been together over the summer but had broken up the second week of school. Tony first heard she was dating some senior guy who lived in her apartment complex, then some self-described "computer geek." When he saw her at the party, Tami had said she missed him very much and wanted to get back together. He was far from wanting to get serious with anyone, but it was still exciting to have a steady girlfriend and to get to have sex. Tony had a few girlfriends in high school and his freshman year of college, but this was the first one who didn't have any hangups about sex. Tami was, as she said, "very comfortable with her body" and had taught him quite a bit between the sheets.

By the end of the day on Monday, Tony had downed several bottles of water and a couple of sports drinks. He had to pee practically once an hour from all those drinks, and it burned worse each time he went. As he fought the snow and ice trekking across campus, he realized he was passing the "Quack Shack"—the University Health Center. I'd better go get checked out, he thought. But what am I going to tell them my problem is? Geez, how embarrassing to say that he had a problem with peeing. Tony had three older sisters who always joked about their tiny bladders and how often they had to stop on road trips to pee. One time, all the siblings had given grief to his oldest sister, Amy, about stopping every five minutes, only to find out when she became ill with fever and chills that she actually had a kidney infection. What if that happened to him? He had a term paper due in one class and a test in another this week. It was certainly not the time to get sick. So, Tony decided to go on into the office and headed over to the scheduling area.

"Um, hi. Can I get an appointment today?" he asked.

"We don't have space left for routine visits today. What kind of problem are you having?" asked the cute girl behind the counter.

"I, uh, think I've got a kidney problem." Tony answered.

"Do you have any fever, chills, nausea, or vomiting?" she asked as she typed into her computer.

"No."

"Back pain?"

"No."

"Burning when you urinate?"

"Yes." There it was, without him having to say it. Phew.

"Discharge?"

Tony flushed from his neck to the roots of his hair. "No!" he hastily replied.

"Okay, then. Our urgent care spots are full for today, but it looks like we can get you in tomorrow morning at ten fifteen. Please come in fifteen minutes early to fill out paperwork. Here is your reminder card." She handed him a small card with his appointment time. "If you get worse during the night, you can call our nurse triage line and they can help. Otherwise, just drink plenty of fluids, and we'll see you back tomorrow."

"Thanks," said Tony. "Well, it can't be that big of a deal, since they're having me come back in the morning," he thought. "Maybe I'll wake up tomorrow and be back to normal anyway." Tony's mind went back to all his tasks for the week ahead. He was totally behind on his paper for English, so he'd actually better head to the library before he went home.

He flushed again when he remembered the girl at the desk asking him if he had any "discharge." How embarrassing. It's not like he had an STD or something. His crazy roommate had actually gotten gonorrhea last year after a particularly wild frat party, and that had been totally different. Now *there* was someone complaining of a "discharge." Joe had whined about catching "the clap" from this loose girl he had slept with. That poor overweight girl was unbelievably desperate for attention from guys. Tony guessed that she had hooked up with half the guys in his frat. He didn't even know her name, but they all called her "Afternoon Delight." Honestly, Tony thought catching something had served Joe right for not being pickier about his sex partners.

Now, a girl like Tami would never give you a disease. She kept herself very together. Tami always looked like she had just stepped out of some fancy magazine, with her clothes always perfectly in style with the current fashions. As he thought about Tami being back in his life, he fished around for his cell phone to give her a call.

"Hey, what's up?" he asked, as she answered the phone right away.

"Not much. Do you want to grab dinner together and then come back to my place to study?" Tami asked.

"Well, I need to get some books at the library, then I can meet you," Tony replied. He laughed to himself as he realized how quickly he had just slipped back into the whole boyfriend role.

After dinner, they went back to her apartment and actually did put in a couple of hours of studying. Unfortunately, Tony needed to get up and go to the bathroom often, and the burning was not particularly getting better. Tony decided to pack up and head back to his room.

"What, you're not staying the night?" Tami pouted. Suddenly, Tony remembered how possessive Tami had always been with his time. It was enough to irritate him into a terse response.

"No, I'm not. I just want to go get a good night's sleep in my own bed," he snapped. Tami looked crushed, and he regretted sounding so harsh. He quickly added, "Honestly, I think I might have a kidney infection or something. It kind of hurts to pee. Have you ever had one before?"

"A kidney infection? Do you mean a bladder infection?" she asked.

"What's the difference?" Tony replied.

"I don't know exactly, but once last year I had to pee all the time, and it kind of hurt went I went. The doctor said it was a bladder infection, and after I took antibiotics for a couple days I was fine. Are you going to the doctor?" she asked.

Tony actually felt kind of relieved to tell her about it. "Yeah, I've got an appointment for the morning. Would you believe that they, uh, they asked me if I had a "discharge"—you know, like I had an STD or something? Isn't that ridiculous?" Tony managed a laugh as he glanced sideways to catch Tami's response. Unfortunately, it appeared this was not what she wanted to hear.

"What is that supposed to mean?" she demanded. "Who were you with while we were broken up?" Tami glared at him across the room.

Tony recoiled, "Whoa...slow down. You were the one dating a bunch of people, but I'm not accusing you of anything. I think I just drank too much beer over the weekend and got a bladder infection or whatever."

Tami chewed on her lip for a minute, then came over and sat down next to Tony. "I'm sorry. I'm sure you're right. When is your appointment?" she asked.

"Tomorrow morning at ten fifteen, right after my English class," Tony replied.

"Oh, good. You at least got a morning appointment. So, do you want to meet me for lunch afterwards? We could grab some sandwiches or something."

"Sounds great." Tony gave her a quick kiss and promised to call her on her cell phone after the appointment.

The next morning, Tony was relieved that it didn't seem to hurt so much when he went to the bathroom. He almost blew off his appointment but decided he might as well go in, since he wasn't completely back to normal. After filling out the mountain of paperwork to check in, he was finally headed back to the exam room. The medical assistant took his weight, temperature, pulse, and blood pressure. Then she began to ask him questions.

"So, what brings you in to see the doctor today?" she asked brightly.

"Heck, don't these people communicate with each other?" he wondered. Tony considered a sarcastic reply, but instead muttered, "I think I have a bladder infection."

"When did your symptoms start?"

"Yesterday morning."

"Do you have burning when you urinate?"

"Yes."

"Any urgency or increased frequency of urinating?"

"Kind of, I guess," he said.

She continued, "Any fever, nausea, or vomiting?"

"No."

"Any discharge from your penis?" she asked without even looking up from her clipboard.

"No!" he exclaimed, feeling the flush return to his face. What was it with these people and "discharge"?

"Any unprotected intercourse in the recent past?" she inquired.

"No."

"Okay, then. Head down the hall to the last door on the left. In the bathroom, there are urine sample cups. Follow the instructions on the wall poster to give us a clean catch specimen, please. Then come back to this room, change into this gown, and the doctor will be in after she looks at your urine under the microscope. Any questions?" She rattled this routine off, as she clearly must have done hundreds of times per week.

Tony actually felt more relaxed as he headed down the hallway toward the bathroom. More relaxed that is, until it hit him that the medical assistant had just referred to his doctor as a *she*. Oh man, a female doctor. Surely she wouldn't have to examine him, would she? What was that part about changing into a gown? He felt his heart racing as he processed this thought.

Quickly he followed the instructions on the wall, wiping off his penis with the special cleanser wipe and then catching his urine in the cup midstream. Of course, it didn't seem to hurt too much now as he peed. Great, I'm here for nothing. Just like taking your car into the mechanic for a funny noise, and it disappears when you've got it at the garage for them to look at. Oh well, if my urine checks out okay, then we shouldn't have to do anything else, I'd suppose. Tony placed the sample in the basket as the sign instructed and headed back to the exam room.

He looked at the gown. Should it be open to the front or the back? He decided to leave his boxers on and wear the coat open to the front like a jacket. He got changed and sat up on the table to wait. Unfortunately, it took a good twenty minutes until the doctor walked in. Plenty of time for Tony to think back over last weekend.

The door popped open and a woman wearing scrubs stepped in. Tony noticed that her arm was in a splint.

"Hi, I'm Dr. Lampert," she said. She looked to be in her late thirties, Tony thought.

"What happened to your arm?" he blurted, shifting the focus onto her.

"I fell off my mountain bike last week and sprained my wrist. Thank goodness it was my left arm, or I could never write my charts," replied Dr. Lampert.

"Cool," Tony replied, then quickly added, "I mean cool that you were mountain biking, not that you got hurt."

The doctor grinned. "No problem, I knew what you meant. Do you bike, too?"

"I love single-track," he affirmed. "My favorite place to ride is the greenbelt behind Mountain Vista."

"No kidding? That's where I fell, past the old bridge, where the switchbacks start."

"And all the big rocks," Tony added.

"Yes, the big slippery rocks," laughed the doctor. "I guess that explains my problem, so let's move on to yours. Your chart says you've had some burning when you pee for the last few days?" she inquired.

Tony felt his pulse racing again. But at least she was looking at the chart, he thought. "Yes. It started yesterday morning, but it seems a little better today," he replied.

"No fever that you were aware of?"

"No."

"And no nausea or back pain?" she asked, taking note of his responses.

"None. Just the burning."

"Got it. Have you had sex with any new partners?"

"Well, I did just get back together with my girlfriend. But no one new." Tony smiled.

Dr. Lampert looked at him intently, asking, "Have you used condoms every time?"

Now Tony was not smiling. "Well, I guess not a hundred percent."

"And you haven't noted any discharge?" she pressed.

"No, despite being asked that a million times here," Tony retorted.

"Sorry, but you'd be amazed how answers sometimes change when they're asked by the doctor," she said, raising an eyebrow.

She put his chart down, stood up, and reached for gloves, which went on easily despite her splint. "Okay. I've already looked at your urine sample, and this doesn't look like a typical urinary tract infection."

"Meaning what?" Tony interrupted.

"Meaning you had some white blood cells, which indicate inflammation, but no bacteria. Therefore, the most common cause of your painful urination would be a urethritis, or inflammation of the tube that carries the urine from your bladder out your penis. Along those lines, we need to go ahead and check you for any sexually transmitted diseases, to see if that's what's causing your symptoms." As she spoke, Dr. Lampert removed a plastic top from a small tube and opened a long paper-covered thing that looked like a Q-tip.

"Go ahead and lie back on the exam table, please." Tony leaned back but stayed propped up on his elbows. Dr. Lampert quickly examined his genitals and then reached for the cotton swab. "Go ahead and lie all the way back. I need to put this in the very tip of your penis, and it tends to sting a bit. It will need to sit there for about thirty seconds to insure a good sample. I have to tell you, I've had guys faint during this test, but from watching it, not from the pain. I really think you'll do better if you just lie back and don't look."

Tony accepted her advice and lay back on the table and looked away. He felt like the test lasted an eternity. It most certainly did sting, but it wasn't as bad as he had anticipated when he first looked at the long instrument.

"All right, you survived," Dr. Lampert said with a smile. Let me step out and let you get dressed. Then I'll be back in to give you a prescription and discuss our game plan."

Tony hopped off the table and grabbed his clothes. He quickly dressed and sat down in the chair. Before he'd even had time to process what the doctor had said so far, there was a knock on the door and Dr. Lampert came back in.

"Okay, Tony. I've got a prescription here for you for a drug called azithromycin. You'll take two five-hundred-milligram pills together at one time today, and that is a complete treatment. You should be feeling better in a couple of days. We'll have your test results back in two to three days. The urine culture takes three days, but I really think that will be negative. To be honest, guys just don't get urinary tract infections as often as girls do, because their urethra is further away from their anus, so the bacteria can't track up as easily to set up an infection. You most likely have a chlamydia infection, which is a sexually transmitted disease. Therefore, if your test comes back positive for chlamydia, your girlfriend will need treatment, too." Dr. Lampert paused a moment, sensing that Tony would have a comment.

"Doctor," he began, "no offense, but I just really doubt this is an STD. Tami is the only, uh, person that I've ever been with, and she's, well, a nice girl." Tony knew that sounded lame, but really, a polished, chic sorority girl like Tami having an STD?

Dr. Lampert took a big breath and let it out slowly. "Tony, I have no doubt that Tami is a great girl. I'm just going to tell you the same rules of life that I see enacted every day, okay?" Tony shrugged his assent.

"Okay, here it is. My three rules to live by: one, everybody has disease. Two, everybody lies. Three, young girls are fertile. Now, let me clarify. Number one, everybody has disease. Nearly ninety percent of adults have oral herpes, which can be transmitted through oral sex, and no one seems to consider this a risk. Many, many people have other diseases like chlamydia or the wart virus but have literally *no* symptoms, so they believe they have no disease, and therefore I guess technically they're not lying, but ultimately they are still passing disease."

She continued, "Most people do know when they have genital herpes, because it hurts. However, it's quite embarrassing to tell someone you're in love with that you've got herpes, so many people frankly just don't. Especially if they haven't had an outbreak in a while. They may be convincing themselves that they just aren't contagious any more, but that unfortunately isn't true."

"As for number three, I've seen more undergrads in here in tears because they're pregnant, even though they were on the pill or using condoms. Condoms break, and inevitably it's the moment the girl is ovulating. The pill is ninety-nine percent effective when it's taken at the same exact time every day, but lots of girls just take it when they wake up or go to bed, which changes by many hours on the weekends versus the weekdays. At the end of the day, my rules stand." Tony just looked at her somewhat disbelievingly.

She continued, "So anyway, the test we just did was for chlamydia and gonorrhea; it'll be back in two days. If the chlamydia portion is positive, you'll already be receiving treatment for that, but if the gonorrhea part is positive, that will require a different antibiotic. If either one is positive, your girlfriend will need treatment. She will have to see her physician in order to be prescribed the appropriate treatment."

Tony sat there a minute. He took the prescription that Dr. Lampert extended to him.

"Do you really think this is chlamydia, or whatever? Wouldn't she know if she had a problem? And what is chlamydia, anyway?" he asked.

Dr. Lampert shook her head as she replied, "No, honestly, most people who have chlamydia are completely asymptomatic—no discharge, no pain, no clue. That's why this disease gets spread so easily. It's actually not hard to treat—just a short round of antibiotics. It's really important to treat it, though, even when people aren't bothered by any symptoms, because down the road, untreated chlamydia infections can cause scarring of a woman's fallopian tubes and therefore cause infertility. It's thought that a majority of infertility is due to this very problem. As for your question about what exactly it is—chlamydia is kind of in between a virus and bacteria. It's bigger than a virus particle, but it lives inside of human cells. That's why it takes a certain type of antibiotic to kill it, one that enters the cells. Does that help?"

Tony sighed, "I guess so. How do you know people have it if they don't know themselves, and they don't have symptoms?"

"Good question. The answer is that any time a woman comes in for her Pap smear and annual exam, which she has to have done in order to get an annual prescription of birth control pills, we ask if she has had any new sexual partners since her last Pap. If the answer is yes, we routinely test for all STDs, including the test I just used on you. You'd be amazed how many come back positive. Speaking of that, I should offer you complete sexual transmitted disease testing since you had unprotected sex. Yes, I know, even just with one person, one time. It's certainly better safe than sorry. We can draw your blood today and check for syphilis, HIV, hepatitis C, and herpes antibodies. If you'd like to do that, I'll grab consent forms for you to sign, and then you just head downstairs to the lab."

Tony put his hand up in the universal sign for stop. "No, thanks. I appreciate what you've said, but I just don't think I need it. I will go ahead and get this antibiotic and take it, but I'll wait until my test comes back before I worry about any other STDs. If it's positive, then I'll come back and get my blood drawn, okay?"

Dr. Lampert shrugged her shoulders and sighed again. "That's your choice, of course. I'll go ahead and write out the lab request and leave it in your chart. Think about it, and think about asking your girlfriend to come in and get tested as well. I encourage you to use condoms if you're going to have sex, both for disease prevention and for extra contraception, even if she's on the pill."

Dr. Lampert finished writing in the chart and on the lab slip. She stood up and opened the exam room door. "You check out down the hall to the right, and they'll direct you to the pharmacy. Let me know if this doesn't take care of your symptoms."

Tony checked out and got his prescription filled at the pharmacy. There was a soda machine in the waiting area, and he grabbed a drink so he could take his medicine. At least they're a reasonable size, he thought, as he popped in the two pills and downed them with the soda. His cell phone rang as he headed out of the building. Yep, right on cue, it was Tami calling to check on him and arrange a meeting place for lunch.

They met at a sandwich shop by the student center. "Well, how did it go? Was it a bladder infection after all?" Tami asked as they sat down with their lunches.

Tony wasn't sure how to answer. "Well, the doctor wasn't sure, but she gave me some antibiotics and took some tests. To be honest, she made a big deal about both of us getting tested for STDs if we were going to...be together."

Tony took a big bite of his sandwich, waiting to see what Tami's response would be. He was afraid she would be offended or defensive. Instead, she was completely unconcerned.

"Well, I get annual checkups for the pill, so I know I'm fine. Did you get everything checked?" she asked.

"Uh, no, not everything. Besides, you know you're the only one I've been with, so if you're clear, so am I." Tony thought back to Dr. Lampert's rules. Was Tami lying, or could she have given him some disease unknowingly? More likely, he just had a bladder infection, and the medicine would clear it up. He cheered up, and they spent the rest of their lunch planning their upcoming weekend.

The next morning, Tony awoke after a good night's sleep feeling great. It didn't hurt to go to the bathroom, and he just generally seemed to have more energy. In fact, Tony pretty much forgot about the infection until Friday morning, when he got a call from the health center. The call came during class, so he checked the voice mail as soon as he got out of the lecture.

"Please call the health center at campus extension 1987; we have your test results available. Please ask for Cindy when you call back," the message said. Why did he suddenly feel so nervous? He dialed the number and asked for Cindy. After several minutes of mind-numbing elevator music, Cindy picked up.

"Hi, this is Cindy. How can I help you?" Tony replied, "Hi, this is Tony Brown, returning your call. You have my test results from this week?"

"Oh, sure, I called you earlier. Just a second while I pull up your results. What's your student ID number?" she asked. "501364," he answered. "Oh, here it is. By the way, are you feeling better?"

"Yes, actually, I feel fine," he smiled.

"Great. Well, your test came back positive for chlamydia, negative for gonorrhea. The doctor's note says here that the antibiotic she prescribed should cover you, but your girlfriend will need to come in to get treated so you don't keep passing this back and forth. Dr. Lampert also left a lab slip in your chart for you to come in and get bloodwork done to check for all the other STDs. You can come straight to the lab, and I'll make sure your slip is there waiting for you, okay? Any questions?"

Tony was momentarily speechless. "So, it's for sure then, that I had chlamydia? Could the test be wrong?" he nearly begged.

"Well, I'm pretty sure it's right." Cindy replied. "It's a DNA test. I hear the doctors say that when it's negative, someone might still have chlamydia, but when it's positive, it's definite. But hey, you already took the medicine that treats the infection, so you don't have to worry. If you want, you can ask the doctor more about it when you come back in. Please make sure your girlfriend comes in to get treated, too, all right?"

"Okay, thanks." Tony hung up the phone. He shook his head, trying to process the information but still unable to believe it. Man, oh man, my first STD. And I hope my very last. Suddenly, everything the doctor said was spinning around in his head. What if he did have another disease that he didn't know about? What if it were HIV, or hepatitis, or that wart virus—gross. He changed directions and headed back over toward the health center. Why hadn't he just gotten his blood drawn while he was there? What was he thinking that day? He certainly wanted his blood drawn now.

And he was the one who said Tami was such a "nice girl." Well, here's one nice girl who had been "nice" to one guy too many. Since he had never had sex with anyone besides Tami, Tony was now completely sure that Tami was the one who had given him this disease. So much for it being a bonus that she didn't have any hangups about sex. That had seemed so cool, but now Tony realized it was not exactly a perk.

The doctor's words echoed in his brain. "Everyone has disease. Everyone lies. Young girls are fertile." He remembered Tami's reassurance that she'd been tested and was "fine." Well, apparently that was before she'd had sex with someone carrying chlamydia and who knows what else. Time for some new testing, Miss Tami, he thought. He dialed her cell, wondering as it rang if he could control his building anger. Luckily for Tami, she must have been in class, because she didn't answer. Tony didn't bother to leave a message.

Although he was extremely teed off, deep down, Tony knew some of his anger was misplaced. He was also really mad at himself. After all, he was the one who asked to remove the condom. How stupid was that? And Tami had been very upfront that she was not a virgin. If Tami had no symptoms, was it really her fault that she gave him an STD? While his bruised ego still pointed the finger at Tami, the logical part of Tony's brain was telling him to go cool off before he made a rash decision about their relationship.

"First things first," Tony decided. "I'll get my blood drawn over at the health center, and make sure we're only dealing with one silent disease. I don't even have all the facts yet," he rationalized. Tony stuffed his phone in his backpack, pulled his hat down to shield his ears from the wind, and hurried off.

7: Lydia

LYDIA PROUDLY SCANNED the boutique, her eyes soaking in all the exquisite clothing. "I'm so glad you finally had a chance to stop by and check out my store. Look at these gorgeous Italian leather jackets," she gushed to her best friend and roommate, Terri. "With my employee discount, I can actually afford one."

"Lucky you," said Terri enviously. "My job at the club certainly wouldn't earn enough to cover it."

"Maybe not, but at least your job keeps you looking great no matter what you wear," Lydia shot back. Both girls laughed. Roommates since their freshman year in college, Lydia and Terri loved to tease each other about their chosen professions. Lydia planned to be a fashion designer, and Terri hoped to own her own fitness center. As recent graduates, they were thankful that each had landed a job in their fields. Terri scored a job as a personal trainer at the busiest fitness center in town. Lydia was the assistant manager at Trixie's.

"Maybe one of your rich clients will start signing up for a bunch of sessions, and you can splurge on something here. Really, though, not everything is superexpensive. Look, how about one of these cute purses?" Lydia said, holding up a brightly colored bag. "Aren't these great?"

Terri slipped the silver straps over her shoulder and modeled the bag for Lydia. "Okay, how does this work with my outfit?" she joked.

Lydia chastised, "Now come on, nothing in here is going to match your sweaty workout clothes and running shoes."

Terri had to agree. "Well, these extra inside pockets for my cell phone and keys would be nice."

"Just getting you to use any purse instead of a backpack would be an improvement," added Lydia. "Well, feel free to look around. Let me know if you see something that you like. I need to get back to the computer and finish a restocking order before I leave for my gynecologist appointment during my lunch break."

"Oh yeah, I forgot you had that today," said Terri. "Glad I came by early, so I didn't miss you."

"I certainly couldn't forget," replied Lydia. "To be honest, I'm actually kind of nervous. I haven't been to the doctor since I got off the pill a few years ago. I'm dreading having a pelvic exam from someone new. You never know how that will be," worried Lydia.

"Oh don't stress, it'll be okay. Didn't you tell me you're seeing Dr. Taylor? I've heard she's great," reassured Terri. "Besides, you don't have anything wrong, do you?"

"Actually, this will be my first time going to the doctor without having some kind of problem," said Lydia.

"So I guess this will make you a real grownup," teased Terri. "Next, you'll be headed to the accountant to pay taxes."

Lydia smiled. "Here's hoping I make enough money to do that."

A few hours later, Lydia found herself seated on the end of an exam table, nervous but pleasantly distracted as she examined the unique style of her patient gown.

"Just toss it on over your head, leaving the sides open like a poncho," the nurse had instructed her.

Lydia's fashion sense was struck by the gown's physical warmth, function, and even whimsy. "Someone found the perfect print for a gynecologist's office," thought Lydia, admiring the bright red ladies' hats, purses, and shoes that adorned the material. From the pastel colors of the waiting room to the beautiful quilt hanging on the wall in the exam room, this practice had obviously put a bunch of effort into aesthetics that would appeal to women. "How nice to have insurance and be able to come here," Lydia mused, starting to relax.

The door opened, and a tall, thin woman wearing black slacks with a black-and-white patterned silk blouse and a stethoscope hanging around her neck strode purposefully into the room. "Hi, I'm Dr. Taylor," she introduced herself, offering a firm handshake.

"Hi, I'm Lydia. It's nice to meet you. My compliments to your interior designer," she added.

"Thank you for noticing," said Dr. Taylor. "My partners and I wanted women to feel as comfortable as possible here. So, I see you're here for a well-woman exam, is that right?"

"Yes," answered Lydia. "I also was thinking about going back on the pill."

"So you've taken a birth control pill before?" asked the doctor.

"I took one for a couple years in high school and college," replied Lydia.

"Do you remember which one?"

"I don't recall the name of it. It was in a compact-style container, like makeup, if that helps," said Lydia.

"Did you have any problems with it?"

"No. I loved it, especially knowing exactly when my period was coming. Also, my periods were a whole lot lighter and I had less cramping," added Lydia.

"So why did you stop taking it?" asked Dr. Taylor.

"Well, I broke up with my long-term boyfriend during my sophomore year of college, and when my prescription ran out, I never went back for an exam to refill it," answered Lydia.

"So what have you done for protection since then?"

Lydia shrugged. "Honestly, I've only had sex a couple times over the last few years, and haven't been serious enough with anyone to think I needed to be back on the pill."

"What has changed now?" asked Dr. Taylor.

"I finally have a job where the benefits include insurance," smiled Lydia.

"That's understandable. Would you like to be tested for sexually transmitted diseases?" the doctor asked. "I try to encourage anyone who has had a new sexual partner since their last Pap smear to be checked for all STDs."

"Why not? If my insurance will cover it, go right ahead," answered Lydia.

Dr. Taylor closed the chart and stood up to examine her. The doctor listened to Lydia's heart and lungs and then asked her to lie back for a breast exam. "On your questionnaire, I saw that you've never had an abnormal Pap smear or an STD," noted the doctor.

"I'd hope not," said Lydia. "Raul and I were both virgins when we started sleeping together."

"Raul was the long-term boyfriend you referred to earlier?" asked Dr. Taylor.

Lydia nodded her agreement. Dr. Taylor was examining her breasts now. "Make sure you do monthly breast self-exams," she was saying. "Start way up here in your armpit, and cover all the breast in circles. I know it may seem like it all feels lumpy, but you're feeling for something that feels hard, or stuck, or just doesn't move with the rest of the breast tissue. Also, look at the skin. If you ever see any redness, dimpling, puckering, or a bruise that you can't explain, you need to come in and let me take a look at it, all right?"

Again, Lydia nodded. The doctor had moved down to her abdomen, and then walked around to the end of the table for the speculum exam. "This may be a bit uncomfortable," said Dr. Taylor, as she positioned the instrument. "Your Pap will be done in a minute. I'm also going to do another test now to check for chlamydia and gonorrhea, which are both STDs. We'll also do a blood test for syphilis, hepatitis C, and HIV." Dr. Taylor finished her exam and stood up to leave. "The nurse will come in to draw your blood, plus I'll have her bring you in some samples of your new pill and explain when to start it. Did you have any other concerns?"

Lydia hesitated, but responded, "I assume that this wouldn't be something you'd deal with, but since you asked, can you tell me what kind of doctor I should see for a painful heel? My right foot has been killing me every time I stand up."

Dr. Taylor glanced over at the chair where Lydia had neatly folded her clothes and set her shoes. "If you're wearing high heels like that every day, it won't matter who you see for foot pain. Try wearing flats, preferably ones that have a rounded toe instead of those pointy ends. I'll ask my nurse to give you a card for a foot specialist, though. You may get dressed, and Jackie will be in shortly."

"Flats with rounded toes? Oh brother," thought Lydia. "That would not be the style statement that Trixie's wants to project. I might as well wear Terri's running shoes. Oh well, maybe I'll check out the foot doctor, anyway." Lydia had barely had time to get dressed when a knock on the door announced the return of the nurse.

"Are you ready?" asked Jackie. "I just need to draw your blood for a few tests, and then I'll explain these," she said, placing a package of contraceptive pills on the counter. She deftly wrapped Lydia's arm with a rubber tourniquet and soon had two tubes of blood collected. "We'll send you the results in the mail if everything is normal," Jackie explained. "If anything comes back abnormal, I'll give you a call."

"Now, here is your birth control. You'll want to start these the Sunday after your next period begins. If your period starts on a Sunday, go ahead and start taking the pills that day. Otherwise, whatever day you have your period, wait until the Sunday of that week to begin the pill pack. We'll need to see you back here during your third cycle on the pill to make sure that everything is working for you and that you don't have any intolerable side effects," instructed Jackie.

"What kind of side effects would that be?" asked Lydia. "I don't remember having any problems with the pill when I took it in the past."

"Then, honestly, you should be fine," said Jackie. "Some people complain about nausea, breast tenderness, or slight bleeding between periods. Usually those things disappear by the third cycle if people hang in there and keep taking the pills at the same time every day. Try hard not to miss any pills, because that not only makes it less effective for birth control, but it makes the side effects worse."

"What about weight gain?" asked Lydia.

"This particular pill isn't bad about fluid retention," said the nurse. "Truly, though, most contraceptive pills do not cause significant weight gain. In controlled studies, roughly a third of the people taking oral contraceptives will gain two to three pounds, and the rest stay the same or even lose weight. Here is our handout on the pill. If you have any more questions that this sheet doesn't cover, feel free to call and ask me. Our number is on the bottom."

"You all seem to have this down to a science," said Lydia, glancing at her watch. "Thanks for getting me in and out so quickly."

"I can't promise it every time, but we certainly try," smiled Jackie. "We'll see you in three months."

A few days later, Lydia and Terri were sprawled out on the couch in their apartment, with a half-eaten pizza sitting in its cardboard box on the coffee table in front of them. Lydia raised her wine glass. "Ah, here's to reliving our college days," she toasted. "When is the last time you and I were actually here by ourselves at the same time? I don't think we've shared a meal in weeks," said Lydia.

"If this is how we eat when we're together, we shouldn't do it very often, or I'd weigh a zillion pounds," said Terri. "What would my clients say if they saw me eating pizza and drinking beer?" she asked, returning the salute with her bottle of Corona.

"Oh, lighten up, Terri. They'd just say you're human. You know we don't eat junk very often anymore. So, catch me up on your life. Do you have any sexy new clients? Remember, you're in charge of my social life now. The last couple guys I picked were pretty lame," said Lydia.

"Especially Mr. 'What's for Breakfast?' don't you think?" taunted Terri.

Lydia groaned. "Come on, don't remind me. That whole night only happened because I'd had such a long dry spell with guys. Surely everyone's entitled to one drunken one-night stand. Oh man, I was sick for two days after that. Truly, I can't even remember his name. What was it, Greg?"

"Gary, not Greg. I wasn't the one doing tequila shots, so I remember quite clearly," said Terri.

"Okay, Gary, whatever. His name is now banished from this apartment, okay? Anyway, we established years ago that you have better taste in guys. Where is your man tonight?"

"Austin is working the late shift tonight. He offered to cover for someone who was sick," answered Terri. "Austin really is a sweetheart. I wish he had a brother for you, because his friends are either taken or definitely not your type. Let me think," Terri said, taking another sip from her beer. "I did start training a cute lawyer this week. He's actually pretty fit already, and he wants to start doing triathlons."

"And he's single?" asked Lydia.

"Absolutely. He was telling me a sob story about how girls don't want to date lawyers, just doctors—oh, hey, that reminds me. I meant to tell you earlier that there's a message from Dr. Taylor's office on the phone for you, asking you to call the office tomorrow. I left the number by the phone for you. How did that go the other day?" Terri inquired.

"It actually went very smoothly. The office was really decorated tastefully, which you know I loved. Everyone was very nice, and I was in and out in less than an hour. I thought the nurse told me they would mail me my results. Oh well, I'll call tomorrow from work and see what's up." Lydia dismissed the call without another thought, and the girls chatted about guys and work until almost midnight.

Lydia dialed Dr. Taylor's office from her cell phone the next morning on her way to work.

"Women's Health Associates, this is Jackie, how may I help you?" chirped the nurse.

"Hi, Jackie, this is Lydia Davis. I was in for a physical the other day, and my roommate said you left a message for me to call yesterday. What's up?"

"Just a second, Lydia, let me grab your chart," said Jackie.

Lydia sipped on her latte as she waited for Jackie to return to the phone.

"Okay, I'm back. Are you still there?" asked Jackie.

"I'm here," replied Lydia.

"Well, Dr. Taylor would like you to stop by this week to see me. Your STD test, which was the swab that Dr. Taylor did along with your Pap smear, came back positive for both gonorrhea and chlamydia, so I'll need to give you a shot of one antibiotic and a prescription for a different one to clear them up. The good news is that your HIV, hepatitis, and syphilis tests all came back negative. Can you come in this morning?"

Lydia looked down at her skirt, where she'd just spilled some of her coffee while listening to Jackie's report. "Sure," she said slowly. "What time did you want me to come in?"

"Actually, I had a late cancellation for ten o'clock, if you can make it here that quickly."

"I'm just a few blocks away, so I'll head right over," said Lydia. She hung up her phone and grabbed for a napkin to blot her skirt. Jackie had been so businesslike, so very matter-of-fact, that Lydia hadn't even questioned what she was saying. "This has to be wrong," thought Lydia. "I don't have any symptoms." Her mind went back and forth, thinking about the couple of guys she'd been with since she broke up with Raul three years ago. "No, this has to be a mistake," Lydia concluded as she parked and headed back into the beautiful office, this time completely oblivious to her surroundings.

The nurse was handing a chart to the receptionist when Lydia checked in. "Great, you got here fast," said Jackie. "Here's your chart, so I can bring you right back."

Lydia stepped through the door that Jackie held open for her and followed the nurse down the hall and into an exam room.

Jackie opened up a cabinet door and began drawing up a shot as Lydia sat down. "So, um, did I understand you to say that I had not one but two diseases?" Lydia asked incredulously. "I mean, there must be a mistake, because I don't have any symptoms at all."

Jackie gave Lydia a sympathetic smile. "Most of the time, that's what we see. Some days it seems like we get as many positive results from our routine screenings as we do from people coming in with complaints of discharge."

"But for two diseases? How is that possible?" asked Lydia.

"I'll give you information sheets on both diseases that will explain more, but these two STDs show up together so often that it's recommended to either test or simply automatically treat for the other infection when one is positive. Think of it as bonus points," Jackie tried to joke. "Seriously, though, consider yourself lucky. With antibiotics, both chlamydia and gonorrhea are completely cured. You certainly can't say that for herpes or warts, and we see those all the time, too." Jackie stepped across the room, helped Lydia to stand up, and prepared her hip for a shot.

"Oh gosh, in my hip? I haven't had a shot there since I was little," Lydia whimpered.

"Sorry, Dr. Taylor believes the hip muscle works better for this shot, with less soreness or swelling than the arm. Ready? This will sting for about a minute," she announced, swiftly delivering the injection.

"It's just hard to believe. I haven't had sex with anyone in over a month, and the time before that was practically a year ago," protested Lydia, reaching down to rub her burning hip.

"Did you use condoms?" asked Jackie.

"Not the one last month. I'm embarrassed to admit it, but I was so drunk that I didn't care. I suppose I'm lucky I didn't get pregnant, on top of everything else. That night was a disaster any way you look at it," said Lydia, shaking her head in disgust.

"I'm sure you'll remember to always use condoms in the future," Jackie said kindly.

"That's for sure," agreed Lydia.

"Well, at least you found out about the STDs. Since these diseases often have no symptoms, a lot of people don't realize they have them until they develop a serious problem like infertility or pelvic inflammatory disease," said Jackie.

Lydia's eyes widened. "Can this make me sterile?"

"Given your time frame, I certainly doubt it. The shot I just gave you was ceftriaxone, and it should completely get rid of your gonorrhea. Here is a prescription for an oral antibiotic, azithromycin. The pharmacist will make you a liquid that you drink all at once, and then your chlamydia will be cured as well. You ought to contact any partners that you've had, so they can go and get tested and treated too. I'm sorry to rush, but why don't you read through these handouts, and then call me if I can answer any more questions for you, okay?"

"Just one last thing, if you don't mind. What are the chances that the test was wrong?" asked Lydia.

Jackie smiled, "This is probably the one statistic that I know, because I get asked that all the time. The test is a DNA probe, with a sensitivity of up to ninety-eight percent and specificity between ninety-eight and ninety-nine percent for each disease. Sensitivity means how often a test detects a disease when it is present, so this test finds the disease when it is there all but two percent of the time. Specificity tells how often people without disease get a negative result, so again this test is very accurate, not resulting in false positives more than one to two percent of the time. The chances of both of your tests appearing positive and actually being wrong is next to nothing. Does that help?"

Lydia shrugged. "It certainly sounds convincing."

"Okay then, you can head back down the hall and check out. I hope to be mailing you the results of your Pap smear," Jackie said, emphasizing the word "mailing."

"One can only hope I've scored enough 'bonus points' already for this visit. No offense, but I'd rather not get another phone call from you," replied Lydia wryly, tucking her information sheets and prescription into her purse and heading out the door.

Lydia slid into her car and pulled out her cell phone. The first call was to Trixie's. "I'm so sorry, but I just accidentally spilled my latte all over my skirt. I need to run home and change, but I'll be there by eleven," Lydia told Marlee, the sales associate who answered the phone.

Tears fell as she drove out of the parking lot and headed back to her apartment. The next call was number one on her speed dial.

"Hey, Lydia, what's up? I've got a client waiting for me at the pool, so I can't really talk right now," said Terri, as she answered her roommate's call. "Lydia, are you crying? What's wrong?"

Between sniffs and a few sobs, Lydia poured out her story. "Remember you said for me to call Dr. Taylor's office? I had to go back in because I caught not one but *two* nasty diseases from my fabulous one-night stand last month. Or at least I can only assume it was him, since I never had any symptoms. I guess it could even be from last year."

"What a jerk! Do you think he knew? Are you going to call him and tell him? And hey, what did you catch? Herpes?" fired Terri in rapid succession.

"No, it was gonorrhea and chlamydia, and at least they're both curable. Who knows if he was even aware that he had anything? As for calling him, the answer is absolutely no way. I don't ever want to see or speak to him again, and frankly, I don't even know if I could track him down."

"Oh, Lydia, you've got to tell him. What if he sleeps with someone else?" Terri protested. "Besides which, Austin mentioned last week that he saw Gary hanging out at his gym. I didn't see any reason to say anything, but I'm telling you now because I know that Austin could ask around and locate him for you."

"Oh, sure, and have Austin plus everyone he asks figure out that I've got STDs? No thanks, Terri. Please, promise me you won't tell Austin. I'll die if anyone finds this out," begged Lydia.

"Look, I've really got to run over to the pool, my client is waiting for me," said Terri, evading a direct response. "I promise not to say anything for now. Let's just talk about it tonight after work, all right?"

"Terri, come on. I trusted you with this information, and I'm asking you not to tell anyone. I'll see you tonight."

"All right," agreed Terri, childishly crossing her fingers behind her back. "Hang in there, and we'll talk later."

Both girls snapped their phones shut, sharing the same thought. "How can she not understand? We'll talk tonight, she'll see the whole picture. I know she'll agree with me."

facts

Chlamydia Fact Sheet

What is it?

- Chlamydia is an atypical bacteria called *Chlamydia trachomatis*.

- Chlamydia can cause "pink eye," upper respiratory infections, and rectal inflammation, as well as infections in the urinary tract and cervix.

How common is it?

- The CDC notes that the reported cases in the United States exceeded one million for the first time in 2006, at 1,030,911 cases.

- Because it is silent up to 70% of the time, chlamydia is largely unreported, and yet it is still one of the most widespread sexually transmitted infections in the United States.

- The CDC estimates that there are at least 2.8 million new cases of chlamydia annually in the United States.

- 2006 CDC data shows that females ages 15 to 19 years old have the highest incidence, at 2,862 cases per 100,000 women, followed by 20- to 24-year-old females at 2,797 cases per 100,000 women.

How do you get it?

- Chlamydia is transmitted through oral, vaginal, or anal sexual contact with an infected partner.

- It lives in semen and vaginal and respiratory secretions.

- Chlamydia can be passed to a baby during vaginal childbirth.

Where on your body do you get it?

- Women usually have infections in the cervix or urinary tract.

- Men get infections in the urethra or epididymis.

- Eye, mouth, and anus infections can occur in either sex.

How do I know if I have it?

- 50% of men and up to 75% of women are asymptomatic, so they only know they have chlamydia if they choose to get tested.

- Tests are conducted from a urine sample or from fluid collected from the cervix or penis with a swab.

- There is no readily available blood test for chlamydia.

- Pregnant women are routinely screened for chlamydia.

- All sexually active women should be screened at their annual exam.

- Infertile couples may discover that past chlamydia infections caused scarring of the woman's fallopian tubes.

- Men can have painful swelling of the scrotum from epididymitis.

What does it look like?

- Normal anatomy or mild red irritation of the cervix or penis, with or without a gray to white discharge.

What does it feel like?

- Usually, people are unaware they have chlamydia.

- If symptoms are present, they include discharge (penile or vaginal) and burning with urination.

- Advanced infection can cause pelvic inflammatory disease (PID), which causes intense pelvic and abdominal pain.

How long does it last?

- Asymptomatic chlamydia infections can silently last for months or years, until treated with appropriate antibiotics (which can happen serendipitously with treatment for an upper respiratory infection).

- Active symptoms can appear within one to three weeks from exposure.

- Symptoms resolve quickly with antibiotic treatment.

Can it be cured?

- Yes. Antibiotics can completely eliminate the bacteria, although they will not remove any damage done by chlamydia (such as scarring of the fallopian tubes).

Can you be re-infected?

- Yes. Prior episodes of chlamydia infection offer no protection. Re-infection is very common, especially when a partner is not fully treated.

- Each subsequent infection with chlamydia significantly increases the risk of long-term consequences.

What is the treatment?

- Antibiotics recommended to treat chlamydia include azithromycin, doxycycline, erythromycin, and ofloxacin.

How about alternative therapies?

- None have been proven to eliminate chlamydia.

Are there long-term consequences?

- 20 to 40% of untreated chlamydia infections will go on to cause pelvic inflammatory disease (PID).

- PID causes scarring and blockage of fallopian tubes, causing an estimated 100,000 women to become infertile each year in the United States.

- Approximately 12% of women are infertile after a single episode of PID, almost 25% after two episodes, and over 50% after three or more episodes.

- PID scarring can also cause ectopic or tubal pregnancy (pregnancy occurring outside the uterus), which is potentially life threatening.

- PID can lead to chronic pelvic pain.

- Newborns exposed to chlamydia through the birth canal can develop serious eye infections or pneumonia within the first few weeks to months of life.

- Women with chlamydia infection are up to 5 times more likely to become infected with the HIV virus if exposed.

When are you contagious?

- Any time you are infected with chlamydia, regardless of symptoms.

- Even while using a condom. Latex male condoms can reduce but not eliminate transmission of chlamydia.

How do I avoid getting chlamydia?

- Abstaining from oral, vaginal, and anal sex will prevent getting chlamydia.

- Consistently using latex male condoms will reduce but not eliminate the risk of getting chlamydia.

- Having sex only in an exclusively monogamous relationship in which both partners have tested negative (or both have been successfully treated) will prevent chlamydia.

If I have chlamydia, how do I avoid giving it to my partner?

- If you have already had sex with your partner, abstain from oral, vaginal, and anal sex until a week after both you and your partner have been treated with antibiotics.

- If your partner has been tested and is negative, and you have not already had sex with him or her, wait one week after you have completed your antibiotic treatment before having oral, vaginal, or anal intercourse.

Can chlamydia be transmitted between homosexual partners?

- Rectal, oral, and urethral chlamydial infections can occur in homosexual male partners.

- Transmission via sex toys theoretically may occur.

- The possibility of female-to-female transmission is unclear, as there is a high incidence of lesbians having past or ongoing heterosexual contact (which makes pure female-to-female transmission rates uncertain).

Frequently Asked Questions

➤ **Is chlamydia is the same as gonorrhea? Aren't they both "the clap"?**
No. The symptoms are often identical, but chlamydia and gonorrhea are caused by different bacteria, so they require treatment with different antibiotics.

➤ **Will penicillin cure chlamydia?**
No. To kill chlamydia, the antibiotic must enter the cell, which penicillin cannot do.

➤ **Can you get chlamydia from a toilet seat?**
No.

➤ **Can you have chlamydia and gonorrhea at the same time?**
Yes, this happens commonly.

Additional Information

American College of Obstetricians and Gynecologists
P. O. Box 96920
409 12th Street, SW
Washington, DC 20090-6920
202-863-2518
www.acog.org/publications/patient_education/bp009.cfm

American Social Health Association
P. O. Box 13827
Research Triangle Park, NC 27709
1-800-227-8922
www.ashastd.org/learn/learn_chlamydia.cfm

CDC-INFO
Centers for Disease Control and Prevention
1600 Clifton Road
Atlanta, GA 30333
1-800-CDC-INFO (1-800-232-4636), 1-888-232-6348 TTY
www.cdc.gov/std/chlamydia/default.htm

MedlinePlus
National Library of Medicine
8600 Rockville Pike
Bethesda, MD 20894
1-888-FIND-NLM (1-888-346-3656), or 301-594-5983
www.nlm.nih.gov/medlineplus/chlamydiainfections.html

GONORRHEA

8: Crystal

CRYSTAL TRIED IN VAIN to find a comfortable sitting position on the exam table. The waistband on her jeans dug into her belly, while abdominal cramps sent spasms of stabbing pain through her torso. Fever and body aches made her break out in a cold sweat, soaking her pink cotton top. "This has to be appendicitis," Crystal moaned to her best friend, Madison.

"At least you look cute in your new outfit," teased Madison.

"Cute doesn't help if I feel like my insides are exploding," replied Crystal.

"Try and use your yoga breathing, Crystal," advised Madison. "Remember how we learned to cleanse our minds with deep breaths and channel our energy?"

"All my energy appears to be focusing on pain, and I'd say it's channeling quite effectively," she snapped.

"Okay, then, at least change into that dressing robe that they left you," suggested Madison tolerantly.

"Quite the fashion statement, isn't it?" mocked Crystal, as she pulled on the patient gown, which was a thin white robe covered in blue polka dots.

"Yeah, right. It would be much cooler if you got to wear scrubs," offered Madison.

Crystal grimaced. "Madi, I don't mean to be such a wimp, but this really, really hurts."

"Hang in there, Crystal, I'm pretty sure you're next," reassured Madison.

"That's what they've been saying for the last hour," whined Crystal.

"I know, but it sounds like the guy in the next section is having a heart attack, best that I can figure." Madison leaned forward, continuing in a conspiratorial low voice, "I heard them talking about an abnormal EKG, and then they asked for the cardiology attending. It's almost like in our acting class last month, when we were performing scenes out of ER and Grey's Anatomy. At least that taught us a bunch of the lingo that they use here in real emergency rooms," said Madison.

"Well, it doesn't need to be Dr. McDreamy for me right now. I'd take any doctor right this minute, as long as they give me something for this pain," responded Crystal through gritted teeth. "This feels like a prison or something. When will they come?" Her eyes searched the tiny makeshift exam room. As if on cue, the curtain slid open, and a tired-looking young guy with rumpled green scrubs and a five o'clock shadow pulled the curtain shut as he sank onto the stool next to the bed. "Hi, I'm Dr. Knight. I understand you're having some abdominal pain today."

"That's the understatement of the century," exclaimed Crystal. "I'm dying, here. Can you please get me some pain medicine? I've been lying here writhing in pain for over an hour."

"I'm sorry, but we've gotten slammed with patients all day long. I need to examine you before I can get you anything for pain, so I'll try and get through your history as quickly as possible, okay?" the doctor said.

"Okay, fire away," consented Crystal.

Looking at her chart, Dr. Knight rattled off, "You're twenty-two years old, with no major medical problems like diabetes, seizures, asthma, or any other chronic illness, right?"

"We think she's got appendicitis, Dr. Knight," interjected Madison.

Dr. Knight looked up, apparently noticing Crystal's friend for the first time. Madison was squeezed between the exam table and the curtain, looking out of place down in the hectic emergency room with her chic dress and perfectly straightened black hair. "I'm sure that's a possibility," he said. Looking back at Crystal, he continued, "Have you had any abdominal surgeries? Appendix, gallbladder, or any gynecological procedures?"

"No," they answered in unison.

"Do you take any medicines on a regular basis?" he continued, noting Crystal's responses in the chart.

"Just my allergy nose spray," Crystal managed to answer.

"And your birth control pill," Madison added helpfully.

"Any allergies to medications?" Dr. Knight continued, focusing on Crystal.

"Penicillin, come on, it's right there on her admissions bracelet," answered Madison, in frustration.

"I'm sorry, but I really need to ask all these questions. I'm trying to help your friend here. Please let her answer," he said, irritation in his voice. "Crystal, what was your reaction to penicillin?"

"My mom says I had a really bad rash everywhere, and they were worried I would stop breathing," she answered.

"Fair enough, that sounds like a true drug allergy," he noted, as Madison rolled her eyes.

"Okay, last set of questions. I see that your last period started ten days ago. Are your periods regular?"

"Usually. I've had some spotting lately," Crystal answered.

"Any chance you could be pregnant?" Dr. Knight asked.

"No, remember, I'm on the pill," Crystal said between held breaths. "And besides, as you read, I just finished my period last week."

"Any new sexual partners within the last couple months?" he inquired.

"Yes, not that I see why that matters," said Crystal.

"Did you use condoms?" he inquired.

"No, she's on the pill," Madison emphasized, as Crystal shook her head no.

"Have you ever had an STD?" asked the doctor.

There was a pause. "I had chlamydia once a couple years ago, but that's all," answered Crystal quietly, looking away from her friend.

"Chlamydia? When did you have that?" interjected Madison, looking at Crystal with surprise. "Where did you catch that?"

"Any vaginal discharge?" Dr. Knight continued, ignoring the comment.

"Honestly, I don't know. I'm just in pain," Crystal complained, also disregarding her friend's questions.

"Okay, let's talk about your pain. Obviously, it's in your lower belly. Is it steady or coming in waves?"

"No, it's not going away. It's steady," she answered.

"Any nausea, vomiting, or diarrhea?"

"A little nausea, yes."

"When did it start?" Dr. Knight asked.

"I've noticed an ache off and on the last few days, but then sometime this afternoon, it really kicked into high gear."

"Let's take a look at you," Dr. Knight said, setting his pen and chart down and standing beside Crystal.

"Finally," muttered Madison under her breath.

"Madison," Crystal warned with a look.

Dr. Knight audibly sighed, "It's all right, I know your friend is just worried about you. Do you want her to stay while I examine you?"

Crystal nodded her assent.

Dr. Knight swiftly examined Crystal's upper body. When he reached her abdomen, he slowed down. He gently examined her belly, starting at the top and moving down.

"Ouch, careful—that really hurts," Crystal protested, as Dr. Knight pressed down on the lower left part of her abdomen.

"The good news is that your appendix is on the other side," said Dr. Knight.

He leaned back and stuck his head out of the curtain. "Is there a nurse available? I'm ready for the pelvic," he called.

A woman came in, pulling a tray. "Okay, sweetie, go ahead and lie back. Is your friend staying?" the nurse asked.

"Yes," Crystal nodded, reaching up for Madison's hand.

When Dr. Knight inserted the speculum, the pain intensified. The nurse handed him several swabs in succession, then Crystal let out her breath as he removed the instrument. When he reached back to perform the second part of the exam, though, Crystal involuntarily cried out.

"That was your cervix, Crystal, the opening to your uterus. Sorry that hurt, but it looks like you've got a pretty bad pelvic infection. I need to do a couple of lab tests and get an ultrasound of your belly."

"So you don't think it's appendicitis?" asked Madison.

"No. She's tender on her left, and the appendix is on the right."

"Then what do you think it is?" Madison pressed.

"Well, I need to make sure it's not an ectopic, or tubal, pregnancy," Dr. Knight replied.

Crystal and Madison were silent, both remembering how their friend Lauren had needed to have surgery the year before for a tubal pregnancy.

"Anyway, once we confirm it's not an ectopic or an abscess, we should be able to treat you with antibiotics and let you go home," he finished.

"Can she get something for the pain?" asked Madison.

"Yes. I'm going to have the nurse start an IV, and we'll give her something to ease up the pain and let her rest," answered Dr. Knight. He took Crystal's chart and slipped out between the curtains. The nurse cleaned up the tray and followed him.

Madison held her friend's hand, trying to comfort her. "Don't worry, I'm sure they'll get you fixed up right away," she said. The two friends remained quiet, Crystal doubled in pain, and Madison listening to the bustling sounds of the ER outside their curtain-rimmed cubicle.

"Now that was what I'd call a 'chandelier' response, wouldn't you agree, Dr. Knight?" said a female voice that Madison thought was the nurse from the exam.

"I'd certainly have to say so. Here's her orders, I'm going to go check on the chest pain in bed nine," answered Dr. Knight.

Another male voice piped up, "What do you mean, a 'chandelier' response, Regina? Does that mean someone thinks they're too fancy for us or something?"

"Go back and study about pelvic inflammatory disease, Ken," said yet another individual. "It's when you do a pelvic and touch the cervix, and it hurts so much the patient jumps up toward the ceiling, you goof." Madison could hear general teasing and laughter following that response.

"It's not very funny when it's you," comforted Madison. They waited for another fifteen minutes or so before anyone came back in to help Crystal. A short-haired brunette entered through the drapes, carrying a tray filled with tubes.

"Hi, I'm Brittany, and I'm here to draw your blood for a few tests," said the perky technician.

"Are you starting her IV to give her some medicine, too?" hoped Madison.

"Nope, that's the nurse's job, but I did see Regina gathering up supplies just now. Is she your nurse?" asked Brittany.

"We're not sure what her name is, but Crystal's nurse is wearing a scrub top with cats all over it, if that helps," answered Madison.

Brittany smiled. "That's definitely Regina. She loves all things cat. I'm sure she'll be right in." Brittany had already slipped a tourniquet around Crystal's arm and was drawing several tubes of blood. She swiftly finished her job, gently rolling Crystal back onto her side, where she stayed tucked in a fetal position. "All done," she announced brightly. "I'll check on your IV for you."

As she left, the drapes flapped open again, and Crystal and Madison looked up expectantly. The curtain was pulled all the way open, and a large cart was wheeled next to the exam table, pushed by a prematurely balding young man in navy scrubs.

"Hi, I'm Dave. Your doctor asked me to do an ultrasound of your abdomen and pelvis," he said, reaching down to plug his machine in an outlet in the wall behind the head of the exam table. "This might feel cold," he advised as he rolled Crystal onto her back, lifting her patient gown and squirting a clear gel on her belly. He pressed the transducer over Crystal's stomach with his right hand and adjusted the viewing screen with his left. Crystal bit her lip to fight her discomfort.

"What are you looking for?" asked Madison.

"Well, this is the gallbladder over here, and I'll be looking at her liver, spleen, kidneys, bladder, ovaries, and uterus," Dave answered.

"Can you see the appendix?" asked Madison.

"Not well, but I can look for any abnormal swelling or fluid in that area," answered Dave, busy with his scan.

Regina, the nurse, stepped up with an IV bag, but retreated, saying, "Oops, sorry, Dave, I'll come back when you're done."

"Wait!" yelled Madison in vain, but the nurse had already left. "We've been waiting forever to get her some pain medicine," she explained to Dave, but he was too intent on his scan to respond.

Just when Crystal thought he must be finished, he began pressing hard on her left groin, making her squirm with pain. "Just hold still for a minute. If you can do that, I'll get done much faster. I know it hurts, but hang in there, okay? I'm hoping to avoid using the vaginal probe. You're thin enough that I might be able to get clear views from on top." That was plenty of information for Crystal. She willed her body to remain as immobile as possible, willing to do anything to avoid any further internal exams. Dave made some adjustments on his machine and seemed to take a bunch of pictures and measurements, too. "Okay, I'm done," he said at last.

"Well, what did you see?" asked Madison, as Crystal turned back to her side and curled up.

"I only take the pictures, and it's up to the radiologist to read them. They really don't like me to say anything," he replied, gathering up his equipment. "You should have the results within an hour or so," he added.

"Things certainly don't move as fast here as they do on television, do they?" Madison tried to joke with Crystal. She craned her neck around the outside of the curtain. "But seriously, I can see your nurse, and now for sure, you're getting that IV."

"Here I am," said Regina, the nurse, brandishing an IV bag and supplies. Again, Crystal was moved onto her back. After a few minutes, the IV was running smoothly. "Okay, sweetie, now I can finally give you some medicine for pain," Regina said, reaching for a syringe. "You may get a funny taste in your mouth or feel burning in your arm, then you'll feel sleepy," she instructed.

"Thank you," whispered Crystal, rolling back to her side.

Nearly an hour later, Dr. Knight came back. "How's she doing?" he asked Madison.

"She's been asleep since they gave her the pain shot," answered Madison quietly. "But I think she's got a fever. She's been shaking some."

Dr. Knight looked at the chart. "Yes, her last temperature was 100.7 degrees. We'll give her some Tylenol when she wakes up."

"I'm awake," slurred Crystal, rolling over and opening her eyes. "What did my tests show? What's wrong?"

"As I suspected, you've got pelvic inflammatory disease, or PID for short," Dr. Knight replied.

"What causes that?" asked Crystal.

"PID comes from sexually transmitted infections, usually gonorrhea or chlamydia. Right now, I can't tell you which one caused yours, but those test results will be available in a couple days. We will go ahead and treat you for both organisms, to cover all the bases. I also sent off tests for other STDs, including HIV, hepatitis C, and syphilis."

"Because they cause PID, too?" asked Madison.

"No, because when you have one STD, you're at risk for the others. We'll have to give you a prescription for an antibiotic that you'll take by mouth to complete your treatment. You need to tell any sexual partners that they should be treated as well, or you can get re-infected easily."

"There's only one right now, and believe me, I'll most certainly let him know," fumed Crystal.

"Don't forget Daniel, from last month," added Madison.

"Thanks for the reminder," said Crystal, narrowing her eyes at her friend.

"I'll have the nurse give you a handout on PID, but the main thing to know is that this is a serious infection, and you need to be certain you complete all your medicine. You are now at higher risk to develop a tubal pregnancy or infertility."

"Are you telling me I can't have kids?" asked Crystal incredulously.

"Not necessarily, but you do need to know that PID can cause permanent scarring and other problems in your reproductive organs, and while the antibiotics will cure the infection, they won't cure any damage that has already happened."

"So what's the chance that I'll be infertile?" asked Crystal fearfully.

"Somewhere between one in five to one in eight women with a single case of PID become infertile," advised Dr. Knight.

"But do you think that I'll be infertile from this? Can you tell? It seems like I've got a pretty bad case, from the pain I'm having," Crystal agonized.

"I'm sorry, but there's no way to predict that," he answered.

"So how long should my pain last?"

"Usually that goes away within a few days of taking the antibiotics. Sometimes it can develop into chronic pelvic pain, but certainly follow up with your regular doctor if the pain lasts more than a week," he concluded.

"Are you going to give me something for the pain?"

"Of course, we'll give you some pain medications in addition to the antibiotics," the doctor reassured.

"I've heard you should douche to clean out vaginal infections. Should Crystal do that?" asked Madison.

"I'm so glad you asked that question," said Dr. Knight. "Absolutely do *not* douche. We think douching increases the risk of PID, likely by forcing what are often silent infections further up the genital tract."

"So women shouldn't ever douche?" followed up Madison, pleased that Dr. Knight had finally appreciated her input.

"In my opinion, basically, no. I would not recommend douching for any woman because we know it disturbs the normal balance of the flora in the vagina, and this can lead to bacterial vaginosis. Even worse, douching can spread a vaginal infection up higher into the reproductive organs. Douching is not only unnecessary, it's potentially harmful."

Both girls nodded their understanding.

"Let's make sure you get your full IV fluids and antibiotics, and then we'll let you check out. Your test results will be mailed to you later this week. Here is a prescription for the oral antibiotic." He looked at Madison. "Can you help your friend get this filled tonight? I want to be sure she gets started on it as soon as possible. We'll give her the first dose here before you leave." Dr. Knight turned back to

Crystal. "I'd like you to follow up with your primary care physician. Do you have any more questions?"

Crystal had closed her eyes, this time to prevent tears. She was an only child, and had long dreamed of raising a big family, filled with as many kids as she could stuff into an extra-large sports utility vehicle. The acting career that she and Madison were pursuing was a fun diversion for now, but the only way theater fit into her long-term goals would be if she were directing a school play. "Focus on the positive," Crystal told herself, putting on her best performer's face.

"No, I don't think so. You said that basically I should have, like, a four-out-of-five chance of this *not* impairing my future fertility, right?" Crystal rephrased with a positive spin.

Dr. Knight smiled. "Yes, as long as you don't get this again, that's correct." He paused for a second, and then added, "Oh, and also assuming that when you were treated for chlamydia, it was discovered right away. The toughest part about STDs is that most of the time, people don't realize they have them."

"But, the doctor said he cured my chlamydia infection back then!" retorted Crystal.

"Well, if you completed all the medicine he gave you, I'm sure it did cure that infection, but you can always get re-infected. There is no immunity, no future protection from having a past infection of either chlamydia or gonorrhea, and both diseases can be present without having any symptoms. The problem is that antibiotics treat the infection, but cannot repair any scarring that might have occurred in your reproductive system. Because your infection may have been silent, going untreated for some time, we don't know if there was any permanent damage. That's part of why it's so hard to make a prediction about your future fertility."

The doctor's words sank into Crystal as he turned to leave. Between physical pain and fear of her fertility, she barely heard his last comments. "I'll write your discharge orders now, but it will probably be another hour or so until your IV is done. A nurse will come unhook you and take care of all your paperwork at that time. Take good care of your friend," he directed at Madison with a wink.

A few minutes passed, both girls immersed in their own thoughts, until Madison broke the silence. "Well, he's not exactly Dr. McDreamy, but I think he really warmed up to me at the end. Do you think he might be interested in me?" she asked hopefully.

All the acting classes in the world couldn't help Crystal mask her shock at her best friend's thought process. "That guy just did a pelvic exam on me. He tells me I might not be able to have kids, and all you can think about is whether or not he's attracted to you?" she exploded. "I hardly think he's looking to either of us for a date," she finished.

"Hey, I'm not the one with a disease," Madison retorted defensively, instantly wishing she could take back those words as Crystal burst into tears. "Oh, gosh, Crystal, I'm so sorry. I didn't mean it like that. It came out all wrong. I know it's not your fault. I'm sorry, and you're right. Everything's going to be okay," Madison blubbered as she wrapped her friend in a hug. "You'll see, it will be alright," she murmured, holding her friend and wishing for the best.

9: Mason

MASON RAISED HIS HEAD from the couch, surveying the scores of empty beer bottles and pizza boxes scattered all over the living room. Two people lay intertwined among blankets and pillows on the floor next to the couch where he had crashed. Spring break this first year in law school was proving to be the best vacation of his life. Ten law school classmates had crammed themselves into a rental van and driven to Florida for its legendary beach parties. Gwen's dad owned this time share right on the ocean, and their crowd filled the small luxury condo.

Mason carefully picked his way to the bathroom, stepping over sleeping bodies and trash along the way.

"Good morning, Mason," yawned a tall, curly-haired brunette dressed only in a t-shirt and underpants, as she headed into the bathroom ahead of Mason. "I'll be out in a second."

"Morning, Gwen," Mason replied. "Take your time."

A few minutes later, Gwen stepped out. "Your turn. Do you want me to start cooking the bacon, if there's any left?"

"That would be great. I'll join you in a minute," Mason replied, trading places with her and wondering how many new "friends" would be joining them for breakfast. "What the?" he glanced down, wondering what on earth could be causing the burning and stinging sensation he was experiencing. He finished urinating and saw a white discharge at the tip of his penis.

Panic set in as Mason washed his hands. "What did I catch? I don't want anyone to know about this. I'd die of embarrassment. Maybe it will go away on its own," he hoped. "Of course, if it gets worse tomorrow, on the twenty-two-hour ride back to Texas, I'll be screwed," he thought. As he washed his hands, he looked at himself in the mirror, shaking his head. "Buck up, buddy. Go find a walk-in clinic and just get this fixed today." Mason shook his hands dry and headed to the kitchen.

"Okay, so what've we got left?" Mason asked, covering for his anxiety by trying to sound carefree. "He and Gwen threw together the remaining leftovers and before long, several other sleepy revelers crawled up to the kitchen table and counter looking for food.

"I can't believe it's already Friday," moaned Jeff.

"I don't want to head back, but I think my liver needs detox," joked Lexie.

"My liver, my head, my stomach," added Sarah.

"Don't forget your sunburned skin," finished Maria.

"Let's hope we didn't do any permanent damage," laughed Jeff.

Mason discreetly knocked on the wooden cabinet in silent agreement.

"Yeah, because remember, what happens in Florida..." started Sarah.

"Stays in Florida!" they chanted.

The chatter picked up as the food disappeared, and soon they were mapping out their plans for their last day. Luckily for Mason, no one had claimed the car yet.

"Hey, Gwen, where did you put the car keys?" Mason asked. "I volunteer to be the responsible one in the crowd. I'll go into town, put gas in the tank, and stock up on munchies for the ride back."

"No, Mason, you should relax. You've been so great about fixing breakfast and cleaning up every day," Gwen looked pointedly around the room, "much better than some people. I don't mind running into town. I have a list of things I want to pick up, anyway. Why don't you head over to the pool or beach. Thanks, though," she said breezily.

Sarah joined in, "Hey, Gwen, I want to come, too. I want to get another throwaway camera so I can take pictures on the beach. I don't want my digital camera to get sand in it."

"Not me," said Maria. "I'm headed straight to the beach. I want to enjoy every last minute of this vacation," she said.

Mason needed the car, and privacy. "Listen, I really don't mind going into town. I'd kind of like to drive around a bit and check out some of the town, since we've really only seen the beachfront. Write up your list for me, and I'll get whatever you need. Since you got us this place, it's the least I can do," he pleaded.

Sarah gave in immediately. "Will you get me a camera? I'll give you the money right now," she said, leaning back to reach for her purse. "Come on, Gwen, let's go scope out the parties down the beach. You know there's going to be a ton of free stuff today since it's Friday, and I want to grab some t-shirts and baseball caps as souvenirs."

Gwen hesitated. "Mason, you're sure you don't mind?"

"Positively," assured a relieved Mason. "You guys make a list of everything we need, and I'll take care of it."

A couple of hours later, Mason parked the van in the parking lot where a sign advertised, "Now Open: 24 Hour Medi-Quick Clinic." The odors of bleach and new carpet permeated the air. "Well, it looks respectable," thought Mason hopefully. Before he spied this clinic, he had passed by a few strip-mall doctors' offices that looked pretty undesirable.

"Good afternoon, how can I help you?" offered the receptionist.

"I'd like to see the doctor," responded Mason.

"Please fill out these forms and then bring them back to me along with your method of payment," said the receptionist. "No problem," assured Mason, in his best courtroom voice. He sat down and began to fill out the forms. Mason was relieved that there were only two other people sitting in the waiting room. That meant he might get seen quickly.

"What a week," Mason reflected. "Who would've thought I'd end up here?" he mused. Surprises the very first night they arrived in Florida had set a tone of decadence for the week. Exhausted from the long drive, the group had staggered into the condo around midnight, everyone lugging their backpacks or suitcases.

"Okay, Sarah and I claim the front bedroom with the ocean view and twin beds for the first night," declared Gwen. "Everyone feel free to fight over the rest," she added, tossing her luggage strap over her shoulder and disappearing into the hallway.

J. R. and Lexie had been snuggling in the van, so it was no surprise when they claimed the back room.

"I'm going to check out the beach scene, so don't wait up for me," said Jeff, dropping his stuff on the floor and appearing to catch a second wind.

"I'll join you," said Rex, always up for a party.

Bonnie looked around and said, "Okay, I'll crash with Mason here on the pullout couch."

Mason had assumed this was a purely platonic sleeping arrangement, until the lights went out. "Ever heard of friends with benefits?" whispered Bonnie seductively, pressing her chest against Mason and wrapping one of her legs across his thighs.

"Seriously?" Mason replied, incredulously.

"Absolutely no strings attached," assured Bonnie. "Let's get spring break started off right," she added, rubbing his chest.

"Why not?" wondered Mason, though he had never had casual sex before. Bonnie's gorgeous green eyes and her ample chest had long tempted him, though her aggressive personality had kept him at bay. He let himself respond to her kisses, but disclosed, "I don't have any, uh, protection, with me, but I'm pretty sure Jeff does. Do you want me to go and get something?"

"No problem, I'm on the pill," Bonnie replied.

The next morning, Mason woke up with second thoughts, worried about what Bonnie might expect. Surprisingly, Bonnie didn't act any differently with him than she had the entire year since they had met, and when she and Kristy brought two guys back to the condo the second night, Mason realized Bonnie definitely wasn't looking for anything more from him.

After that, Mason had completely relaxed and partied hard along with his classmates. J. R. had ceremonially distributed a handful of condoms to the three other guys the first morning, encouraging them to practice safe sex. Mason was surprised to find himself needing one of them, thankful for the protection when he hooked up with a local waitress named Sonia later in the week.

"So which girl gave me this?" he wondered, though it was more likely to be Bonnie, because they hadn't used a condom.

"Mason?" said a young man in white scrubs from the doorway, interrupting Mason's thoughts.

"That's me," he answered.

"I'm Jaime, the medical assistant here," said the man. He weighed Mason, took him into an exam room, and charted all of Mason's vital signs. "So you've noticed a discharge?" he asked, reading the form Mason had filled out.

"Yes, just today," answered Mason.

"Any burning?"

"Only when I urinate," replied Mason evenly.

"Have you had unprotected sex with any new partners recently?"

Embarrassed, Mason limited his answer to a monosyllabic yes. In his mind, however, he added, "Which I know was incredibly stupid. In the heat of the moment, I just didn't think." Admitting that he chose not to use a condom felt completely ignorant.

"Okay, the doctor will be in to examine you shortly," said Jaime. "Please get undressed from the waist down and have a seat on the exam table."

Mason followed the directions, covering himself with the paper drape.

The door popped open. "Hello, I'm Dr. Martinez," said a young Hispanic man, impeccably dressed in pressed khakis, a white button-down shirt, and festive tie, topped with a starched white lab coat. "Are you down here for spring break?"

"Yes," clipped Mason, not feeling particularly social.

The doctor perused his chart. "Looks like you might have had a bit too much fun," he commented. "When did you first notice any symptoms?"

"First thing when I urinated this morning," replied Mason.

"No fever, nausea, or rash?" asked the doctor.

"Just the discharge and stinging," said Mason.

"Let's take a look, then," said Dr. Martinez, setting down the paperwork. "Go ahead and lay back." The doctor examined him, noting, "I see the discharge you were talking about. You've also got some swollen lymph nodes here in your groin, which is expected, but I don't see anything else. I'll do a couple tests to confirm it, but it looks like you have gonorrhea. When was your contact with a new partner?"

"Sunday night," replied Mason, and then after a brief pause, sheepishly added, "or possibly Wednesday night, but that time I used a condom."

"Either one could be the right timing, but it's more likely from the time that you didn't wear a condom. When gonorrhea is symptomatic, it can appear as early as two days after exposure, although it can be as much as thirty days later," the doctor explained, as he took a long, skinny package from his coat pocket. He opened it up, removing a test tube and a swab. "This will sting a bit," he informed Mason. "We test for both gonorrhea and chlamydia, because those two diseases like to travel together."

He took a sample of the discharge from Mason's penis and then broke off the tip of the swab in the test tube and capped the tube. Then he removed one more swab from a wrapper and took another sample of the discharge. "I'll look at this one under the microscope right now," he said. "Go ahead and get dressed, and I'll be back in a couple of minutes."

Mason quickly pulled on his underwear and jeans, relieved to be dressed again. In a few minutes, Dr. Martinez returned.

"What I saw under the microscope was consistent with gonorrhea. There were a bunch of white blood cells, which shows inflammation. Your definitive test for chlamydia and gonorrhea we send out to the lab."

"When will I get the results?" Mason asked.

"We should have them on Monday," replied the doctor.

"Monday?" Mason repeated, alarmed.

"Don't worry, I'll give you antibiotics today. The test is a confirmation, in this case primarily so you can inform your two partners that they need to be treated. Actually, you should tell anyone you've had intimate contact with over at least the past month."

Mason felt foolish, but for some reason he didn't want the doctor to think he slept around indiscriminately. "Believe me, these two are it. I hadn't slept with anyone in over a year prior to this week."

"Busy week, then. Spring break can be dangerous," commented Dr. Martinez. "When you get back home, you need to go to your regular doctor and get tested for all STDs. I can do it here if you'd like, but usually people want to be sure their insurance will cover it, because it's pretty expensive."

"What else do you think I need to be tested for?" asked Mason.

"Blood tests are available for HIV, hepatitis C, syphilis, and herpes," answered Dr. Martinez.

"I can't imagine Bonnie would have anything like that," Mason mused out loud, picturing his confident, assertive classmate.

"Think about it, Mason," said the doctor, "all STDs are basically passed the same way. If you have one, you're at risk for the others. Don't kid yourself that nice girls, or nice guys for that matter, won't have bad diseases. Hopefully all you've caught is one or two bacterial illnesses, both of which we can cure."

"How are you going to treat me?" asked Mason.

"We're going to give you a shot of one antibiotic and a single dose of two pills of another. The shot will cover gonorrhea, and the pills will treat chlamydia."

"Is the shot penicillin? They say it cures everything, but I think I'm allergic to it," said Mason.

"Actually, about the only disease that penicillin still cures within the STDs is syphilis. Everything else is resistant. The shot we're going to give you is ceftriaxone, which is a cousin of penicillin. In theory, there's about a ten percent chance of you also being allergic to it if you have a true penicillin allergy, but in practice we rarely see that. What was your symptom of allergy to penicillin?"

"I really don't know. My mom said I got a rash or something

when I was little, and they thought it might be an allergic reaction to penicillin," said Mason.

"I think you'll be fine, then. Do you have any questions for me?" asked the doctor.

Mason thought for a minute. He had tons of questions, though not all were for the doctor. "Knowledge is power," they say, so he'd better start arming himself. "How common is this? Is this what they call 'the clap'?"

"Yes, 'the clap' traditionally refers to gonorrhea, and it is more common than you'd think. Chlamydia is the most common bacterial STD, with 2.8 million infections per year. Gonorrhea is the second most common one, at roughly seven hundred thousand new cases per year. Trichomonas is the most common nonviral STD overall, at over seven million new cases per year, but it doesn't usually cause a visible discharge," instructed Dr. Martinez.

"Once I take the antibiotic, then am I completely cured? Also, does this make me immune in the future?" Mason asked.

"Yes, you should be cured. I doubt you've had it long enough to cause permanent damage. Some cases can lead to infertility in guys, but that's usually because guys are asymptomatic, not realizing they're carrying around a silent infection for years," the doctor explained. "However, you will not be immune to getting it again. These antibiotics will treat this infection, but you can catch it again."

"How often do girls know they have this disease?" asked Mason, wondering about Bonnie.

"Somewhere between twenty and forty percent of women have no symptoms. It's important for them to be diagnosed so they don't develop scarring and other problems that lead to infertility. Obviously, you need to let your two partners know that they should be treated," concluded Dr. Martinez.

"Can you just give me extra medicine to treat my, uh, partners? I mean, I know you wouldn't hand me a shot to give someone, but are there pills available that would work just as well?" asked Mason.

"Not in Florida. I saw from your paperwork that you're in law school, so you might find this interesting. If I were to give you medicine for you to deliver to anyone you have been intimate with, that's called expedited partner therapy, or EPT for short. The idea is that we would be more successful in cutting down on the spread of STDs if we made treatment more accessible that way. The downside is that we would be treating a patient we've never seen, who could have underlying medical issues or drug allergies that could create a problem. Since 2006, thirteen states prohibit EPT, and Florida is one of them. Texas, I believe, allows it under certain circumstances, but right now I'm afraid you're out of luck."

"I guess I feel badly about the second girl, in case I passed this on to her," Mason admitted.

"Send her over, and we'll take care of her," said Dr. Martinez cheerfully. "Anything else, or are you ready for your medicine?"

"One last question. I've been living in a three-bedroom condo with anywhere from ten to twenty people on a given night this week. How contagious is this? Could we have passed it to one another in the bathroom?"

"Only if you were having sex in there," Dr. Martinez replied with a chuckle. "These diseases are not passed by toilet seats, despite popular myths. STDs are transmitted by intimate contact, either by direct genital contact, oral-genital contact, genital-anal contact, or sharing sex toys. If you stayed clear of those, you're not guilty of putting your roommates at risk." Dr. Martinez stood up to leave. "My assistant, Jaime, will be back in with your medicines, and we'll call you on Monday with your test results. Your symptoms should clear up quickly over the next couple of days. By the way, since this is likely your last night here, I should tell you that it's okay to drink alcohol with these antibiotics, but on general principle, I'd limit it to a couple drinks. Good luck."

"Thanks," said Mason.

Jaime came in and smoothly delivered the shot, which stung like crazy, and watched while Mason swallowed two capsules. "Okay, you're free to check out," instructed Jaime.

"Free" might not have been the most appropriate word, thought Mason. Back in the van, although several hundred dollars lighter, he breathed a sigh of relief. "At least I'm treated," Mason concluded. He glanced at his watch, which showed 2:30 p.m. "Okay, I've got time to get the groceries and gas, and I can slip into Dos Margaritas and find Sonia." He knew she'd be upset, but if he left Florida without telling her, his conscience would never let him rest. Mason planned to spend his last night out on the beach, simply enjoying the waves, maybe a couple beers, and definitely some solitude.

"How should I confront Bonnie?" Mason wondered, as he began to deliberate the best approach. "In fairness," he thought, "Bonnie may have no idea that she has this disease. Knowing her, I'd better wait 'til I have proof from the tests." In mock trials at school, Mason had seen Bonnie rip apart arguments that lacked substance, and by no means did he want to face her unarmed. On the other hand, Mason realized there was a reasonable chance that on this, the last night of spring break, Bonnie could become a repeat offender. "I'll actually be an accessory if I don't tell her today," he realized.

Mason started the van and headed out of the parking lot in search of the nearest grocery store. The debate persisted onward in his head, bringing in new factors. "What if she makes a huge scene and accuses me of giving this to her? What will everyone think? Who will they believe?" Bonnie could be like a pit bull, never letting go once she got her teeth in something, and Mason had no desire to spend nearly twenty-hour hours in a van listening to her hold forth.

"What if I hear she also slept with Jeff or J. R.? Should I tell them?" Mason's internal arguments continued until his legal intellect was exhausted. "I guess the jury's still out on this one," Mason conceded. "I don't know what I'm going to do."

facts

Gonorrhea Fact Sheet

What is it?

- Gonorrhea is a sexually transmittable disease caused by the
  Neisseria gonorrhoeae bacteria.

How common is it?

- CDC 2006 Surveillance Report statistics:
  - An estimated 700,000 people are infected each year in
    the United States, although only half of those cases are
    reported, partly because some people are asymptomatic.
  - Gonorrhea is the second most commonly reported bacteri-
    al sexually transmitted disease in the United States (behind
    chlamydia).
  - 20- to 24-year-olds have the highest rate of gonorrhea at
    527.5 cases per 100,000, which is more than 4 times the
    national average (120.9 per 100,000).

- Female 15- to 24-year-olds have more than 605 cases per 100,000, while men 20 to 24 years old have 454 cases per 100,000.
- African Americans have much higher rates than Caucasians or Hispanics (658 per 100,000 vs. 37 and 77 per 100,000, respectively).

How do you get it?

- Gonorrhea is transmitted through oral, vaginal, penile, or anal sexual contact with an infected partner.

- Ejaculation does not need to occur to transmit the disease.

- Gonorrhea lives in semen and in vaginal secretions.

- It can be passed to a baby during vaginal childbirth.

Where on your body do you get it?

- Women usually get infections in the cervix or urinary tract.

- Men get infections in the urethra or epididymis.

- Eye, mouth, and anus infections can occur in either sex.

- Gonorrhea can spread to the blood or joints.

How do you know you have it?

- Many people are asymptomatic, so they only know they have gonorrhea if they choose to get tested.

- Men typically have penile discharge, along with burning with urination, and can also have painful swelling of the scrotum from epididymitis, which can lead to infertility.

- Women can have vaginal discharge, spotting between periods or after intercourse, pelvic pain, or painful urination.

- Both men and women can develop rectal symptoms, including itching, pain, discharge, bleeding, or pain with bowel movements.

- Tests are conducted from a urine sample or a sample of fluid from the cervix, penis, or throat, depending on location of symptoms. There is no readily available blood test for gonorrhea.

- Pregnant women are routinely screened for gonorrhea.

- All sexually active women should be screened at their annual exam.

- Infertile couples may discover that past gonorrhea infections caused scarring of the woman's fallopian tubes.

What does it look like?

- Normal anatomy or mild red irritation of the cervix, penis, or anus, with or without a white, yellow, green, or bloody discharge.

What does it feel like?

- Often, people are unaware that they have gonorrhea. An estimated 20 to 40% of women and 10% of men have no symptoms.

- If symptoms are present, they include discharge (penile or vaginal) and burning with urination.

- Women can notice vaginal bleeding between periods.

- Advanced infection can cause pelvic inflammatory disease (PID), which causes intense pelvic and abdominal pain, vaginal bleeding, vomiting, or fever.

- Rectal disease produces discharge, itching, soreness, bleeding, or painful bowel movements, or may be asymptomatic.

- Testicular pain comes from epididymitis.

How long does it last?

- Gonorrhea infections can exist silently for an unknown period of time until treated.

- Active symptoms can appear within two days to several weeks from exposure.

- Symptoms usually resolve quickly with antibiotic treatment, unless there is antibiotic resistance.

Can it be cured?

- Yes. Antibiotics can completely eliminate the bacteria, although they will not reverse any damage done by gonorrhea (such as scarring of the fallopian tubes or epididymis).

- However, there is a great deal of antibiotic resistance, especially in Asia and the United States, with more developing each year. This means that gonorrhea is becoming more difficult to treat as it becomes resistant to standard antibiotic therapy.

Can you be re-infected?

- Yes. Prior episodes of gonorrhea infection offer no protection. Re-infection is very common, especially when a partner is not fully treated.

- Each subsequent infection with gonorrhea significantly increases the risk of long-term consequences.

What is the treatment?

- Antibiotics recommended to treat gonorrhea in the past have included ceftriaxone, cefixime, ciprofloxacin, ofloxacin, and levofloxacin, usually in a single dose. As of April 2007, the CDC has changed its guidelines and no longer recommends any of the fluoroquinolones listed above (ciprofloxacin, ofloxacin, and levofloxacin) due to advanced drug resistance of gonorrhea.

- The CDC recommends testing or directly treating for chlamydia at the same time (with different antibiotics) because the two diseases are commonly both present.

- Notify anyone you have had sexual contact with in the last two months, so their doctors can treat them for gonorrhea regardless of whether or not they have symptoms.

How about alternative therapies?

- None are proven to eliminate gonorrhea.

Are there long-term consequences?

- Estimates vary, but 10 to 30% of untreated gonorrhea infections in women will go on to cause pelvic inflammatory disease (PID). Gonorrhea and chlamydia are the primary causes of all PID.

- PID causes scarring and blockage of fallopian tubes, causing an estimated 100,000 women annually to become infertile.

- PID scarring can also cause ectopic or tubal pregnancies (pregnancy occurring outside the uterus), which is potentially life threatening.

- PID can lead to chronic pelvic pain.

- Newborns exposed to gonorrhea through the birth canal can develop throat infections or serious eye infections leading to blindness if not treated within the first few weeks of life.

When are you contagious?

- Any time you are infected with gonorrhea, regardless of symptoms.

- Even while using a condom. Latex male condoms can reduce but not eliminate transmission of gonorrhea.

Can gonorrhea be transmitted between homosexual partners?

- Male homosexual transmission occurs via anal and oral sex.

- Female homosexual transmission is theoretically possible but not proven.

How do I avoid getting gonorrhea?

- Abstaining from oral, vaginal, and anal sex is 100% effective.

- Consistent and correct use of condoms will prevent transmission of gonorrhea from a male to a partner, as long as the condom does not break.

- Use new condoms for each partner with any shared sex toys, or preferably, do not share sex toys.

- Female barrier methods and spermicides are less effective than condoms but do decrease transmission somewhat.

- Have intercourse only within a monogamous relationship in which both partners have tested negative for gonorrhea.

If I have gonorrhea, how do I avoid giving it to my partner?

- If you have had no sexual contact yet with your partner, abstain from oral, vaginal, and anal sex until you complete your antibiotics and any symptoms have resolved.

- If there has been any prior sexual contact with your partner, abstain from oral, vaginal, and anal sex until *both* of you have completed antibiotic therapy and any symptoms have resolved.

Frequently Asked Questions

➤ Is gonorrhea is the same as chlamydia? Aren't they both "the clap"?
No. "The clap" typically refers to gonorrhea. The symptoms of both diseases are often identical, but different bacteria cause chlamydia and gonorrhea, so they require treatment with different antibiotics.

➤ Will penicillin cure gonorrhea?
No. Currently, the only class of antibiotics recommended to reliably kill gonorrhea is the cephalosporin class, which is a cousin of penicillins.

➤ Can you get gonorrhea from a toilet seat?
No.

➤ Can you have chlamydia and gonorrhea at the same time?
Yes, this happens commonly. If you have one, you should be treated and/or tested for the other one.

➤ Can you get gonorrhea from douching?
No. However, douching can cause pelvic inflammatory disease (PID) by forcing vaginal infections (often silent) up into the cervix and into the uterus or fallopian tubes.

Additional Information

American College of Obstetricians and Gynecologists
P. O. Box 96920
409 12th Street, SW
Washington, DC 20090-6920
202-863-2518
www.acog.org/publications/patient_education/bp071.cfm

American Social Health Association
P. O. Box 13827
Research Triangle Park, NC 27709
1-800-227-8922
www.ashastd.org/learn/learn_gonorrhea_fact.cfm

CDC-INFO
Centers for Disease Control and Prevention
1600 Clifton Road
Atlanta, GA 30333
1-800-CDC-INFO (1-800-232-4636), 1-888-232-6348 TTY
www.cdc.gov/std/Gonorrhea/default.htm

MedlinePlus
National Library of Medicine
8600 Rockville Pike
Bethesda, MD 20894
1-888-FIND-NLM (1-888-346-3656), or 301-594-5983
www.nlm.nih.gov/medlineplus/gonorrhea.html

TRICHOMONIASIS

10: Meredith

SWEAT DRIPPED DOWN MEREDITH'S back as she jogged toward the final turn at Town Lake. "With weather this nice, I know I can stay motivated to keep exercising and lose these 'freshman fifteen' pounds I put on last year," she thought. Too many pizzas and beers, plus her love of Mexican food, had piled on the calories. Who can resist chips and queso? Not Meredith, especially last semester when she was nursing a broken heart. "No sense in dwelling on the past," Meredith chastised herself. She pushed her stride into a sprint for the last half mile, clearing her mind of negative thoughts and visualizing her healthier body.

The next morning, Meredith was less optimistic as she sat in the waiting room to see her primary care physician. She seemed to be coming here way too often. This was the fourth time in about six months that she had come in for one problem or another. Does your body's warranty run out at twenty? Her mom always joked that it was at age forty that everything started to fall apart. If so, Meredith was two full decades early.

It had all started last October, when she caught strep throat after a Halloween party. It was a "famous couples" costume party, and she and her boyfriend Marc had gone as Superman and Lois Lane. Unfortunately, later that night, she had seen her Superman making serious moves on Olive Oyl—where was Popeye when you needed him? Meredith and Marc had broken up the next day, and on top of being depressed, Meredith had developed a fever, chills, and a horrible sore throat.

She had come in to see Dr. Messer the next day, and after a quick swab from her throat, the doctor had told her she had strep throat. She even agreed to get a shot of antibiotics, rather than pills, because it was so painful to swallow. The sore throat disappeared pretty quickly, but then around a week later, she noticed a discharge on her underwear, and sometimes it burned when she urinated. Meredith wondered why on earth strep throat would cause a problem "down there." That time, Meredith didn't see the doctor. She called in and spoke with the nurse, who gave her the option of taking over-the-counter medicine to treat her symptoms. The nurse explained to her that women always have both yeast and bacteria in their vaginas, and when you take an antibiotic like she had, it kills off bacteria in all parts of your body, not only in your throat. With the vaginal bacteria killed off, the yeast can overgrow, and you get a discharge. This explanation made sense, and anyway, Meredith was not anxious to have a pelvic exam besides her yearly checkup. Her symptoms improved with the yeast treatment, but roughly a month later, she again started having irritation and burning when she went to the bathroom.

That time, Meredith did go back in to see the doctor. It was right after Thanksgiving break. Meredith had been home in Omaha, wearing several layers of clothes to keep warm, meanwhile peeing all the time. She didn't want to say anything to her mom about her symptoms, partly because their family doctor back home in Nebraska was a man, and Meredith would rather die than see a male doctor for any problem that might require a pelvic exam. Of course, Meredith also was afraid that if she told the doctor that she'd had sex, her mother might somehow find out. Instead, she dealt with her symptoms and hid her discomfort for a few more days. She couldn't wait to get on the plane and return to college!

[136]

Back at school, when she went to see the doctor, they skipped the pelvic anyway. Since she was complaining of urinary symptoms, the first thing the medical assistant did was to collect a urine sample. They "dipped" the urine (which means they dipped a test strip of paper into the urine that checks for sugar, blood, white blood cells, and pH levels). Then the urine was looked at under the microscope. Apparently, Meredith's urine had "loads" of white blood cells in it, so they were able to treat her for a urinary tract infection without needing to do a pelvic exam. She took a course of antibiotics, which seemed to be the most enormous pills Meredith had ever seen. To be honest, the drugs didn't really make all of her symptoms go away, but with all the activities of the holidays, Meredith ignored it and went about her life.

Close to Valentine's Day, Meredith once again began having symptoms. By now, she had tried all the home remedies for bladder infections. She was drinking tons of cranberry juice and water. So much, in fact, that Meredith had to pee constantly, even during the night. There was no way she could get any decent studying done with all this lack of sleep and interruptions during the day for bathroom breaks. Meredith went back to the doctor's office.

Again she gave a urine sample, and again it contained white blood cells. Dr. Messer asked about any vaginal symptoms and whether or not she was sexually active. Meredith laughed and said she had sworn off guys since getting dumped by Superman last year, and no, she didn't have any vaginal discharge. In truth, she had noticed a vaginal discharge off and on over the last several months, but that week it seemed to be gone. "Since you had a urinary tract infection fairly recently, I'm going to give you a stronger antibiotic this time, plus we're going to culture your urine to identify specifically which bacteria you are infected with," said Dr. Messer. At least the new antibiotic was a smaller tablet than the medicine she'd taken last time. Unfortunately, three days later the nurse called Meredith with some disappointing news.

"Hi, Meredith, how are you feeling?" asked the nurse.

"Well, a little better, I guess," answered Meredith.

"I'm glad you're feeling better, but we got your urine culture back, and it actually was negative," said the nurse.

"Negative? What does that mean?" asked Meredith.

"It means you didn't have a bacterial urinary tract infection, so you can stop taking the antibiotic we prescribed. Drink plenty of water, and if your symptoms don't go away completely, then please schedule an appointment and come back in and see us, okay?"

"All right, although I can't possibly drink any more than I've been doing already. What else could it be?" asked Meredith.

"Maybe we need another urine culture, or perhaps you have a vaginal infection," suggested the nurse. "Be sure to follow up with us if you don't get better, okay?"

So, here it was, around ten days later, and Meredith decided she'd better come back and get things checked out. Now that she thought about it, she had really had some irritation off and on for nearly five or six months. She kept thinking that maybe it had something to do with her menstrual cycle, because it seemed to get worse after each period. Oh well, hopefully this time we can figure this out, she thought.

The medical assistant handed her a gown and a sheet and asked her to get changed so the doctor could examine her. Meredith shed her clothes, put on the gown, and climbed onto the examining table. She was happy that they didn't have the temperature super cold today. While she waited, Meredith flipped through the school newspaper and was excited to see one of her favorite groups scheduled to headline a local fundraising concert next weekend. She was scanning the ad for details when Dr. Messer walked in.

"Hi. I'm sorry you're still having problems. Let's see if we can figure out what's going on with you, okay?" she asked. "Now, what symptoms are you having?"

"Well, it's nothing awful, but I keep having irritation when I pee. It comes on for a few days, then goes away for a week or so, then comes back. Sometimes it's worse than others, but I don't understand why the antibiotics aren't working, and why the nurse told me it doesn't look like I have a bladder infection," said Meredith.

"Well, that's what we need to figure out," said the doctor. "Let me ask you a few more questions before I take a look at you. Have you had any fever?"

"No."

"Any back pain?"

"No."

"Nausea or vomiting?"

"Nope."

"And have you had any vaginal discharge or discomfort?" Dr. Messer asked.

Meredith paused for a moment. "You know, I have had some off and on, but I'm not sure if it has happened when I've had the burning when I pee, if that matters."

"When is the last time you had sex?"

"Gosh, a long time ago—basically Halloween," Meredith replied. "That's too long ago to do anything, isn't it?"

"Not necessarily. Did you use condoms?" the doctor asked.

"Well, not always," Meredith admitted.

"Sometimes sexually transmitted diseases can cause urinary symptoms, too. Let's go ahead and do a pelvic exam on you and we'll check for that as well, okay?" said Dr. Messer. "If that is what is going on, it would certainly explain why the antibiotics didn't cure your bladder infections."

"Okay, I guess," said Meredith, lying back and scooting down the table. Mercifully, Dr. Messer was speedy, and the exam passed without much discomfort.

"All right. I took a sample of your discharge during the exam, and I'm going to go and look at it under the microscope while you get dressed. I'll be right back," said Dr. Messer as she stepped out of the room.

Meredith got dressed and sat down in the chair next to the table. She was about to get out her economics notes to study when there was a quick knock on the door and Dr. Messer came back into the room.

"Well, we've got your answer, and we should definitely be able to clear up all your symptoms," the doctor said with a smile.

"What is it?" Meredith asked.

"You've got something called trichomoniasis, or 'trich' [pronounced "trick"] for short. It is a sexually transmitted disease, and either the second or third most common one in the United States, depending upon whose statistics you use. It can take anywhere from one week to six months to show up, and it is often completely asymptomatic, so it's likely that you've had this as the cause of your intermittent symptoms for the last several months. The previous antibiotics you took can't kill it but often will suppress the symptoms for a while. Trich is a little single-celled protozoan that is about the size of a white blood cell."

She pulled out a handout from her clipboard and pointed to a picture of the protozoan. It looked like a fat triangle with a curly tail to Meredith. "It can be simple to see under the microscope if you look immediately, when they are still swimming. Unfortunately, if the slide sits out for several minutes and dries out, it's much more difficult to pick them out if there are only a few mixed in with a bunch of white blood cells, because they're the same size and shape as those white blood cells. Today, as soon as I put your slide on the microscope, I saw three or four of them spinning around the minute I looked through the lens. They say that it is only identified about half the time by using a microscope. It can also be identified by a culture, but not the type of standard culture that we use for urine, which is why we missed it before."

"Oh," said Meredith, still a bit confused.

"One concern we have with trich is that it is often associated with other STDs. Some studies have shown that trich makes it easier to get other STDs, particularly HIV."

"What?" exclaimed Meredith. "I go from having a bladder infection to HIV?"

"Listen, I'm not at all saying that you have HIV, or any other STDs, but that having trich can increase the chance. With any STDs, including trich, we suggest testing you for all STDs. I already did a swab for chlamydia and gonorrhea when I did your exam, and now we can draw your blood for HIV, syphilis, and hepatitis C. We'll hope that you only have trichomonas, but it's important to be sure."

"Okay, okay, that seems reasonable. Sorry I panicked there for a minute, but honestly, I wasn't expecting this to be an STD when I thought it was all about my bladder. Not to mention, I've only had sex with one guy in my whole life, and we broke up last October... it's not fair," said Meredith, her eyes filling up with tears.

"I'm sorry," said Dr. Messer. "STDs are certainly never 'fair.' The fact that you've only been with one guy definitely decreases your risk of having other STDs."

"Well, clearly Marc gave me this, so who's to say he didn't give me something else?" Meredith asked.

"You're right, and that's why we're going to test you for everything, to be sure. Anyway, the good news is that we definitely can cure trich. Here is a prescription for an antibiotic called metronidazole. You take one pill twice per day for a week. There is a single-dose method too, but I find that it tends to cause more side effects. Make sure you don't drink any alcohol at all while you are on the medicine, because that can cause a miserable reaction with severe nausea and vomiting. Of course, your ex will likely need to be treated too, so he doesn't spread this to anyone else."

"Um...how does that work? Do I give you his name, and someone calls him?" Meredith asked hopefully.

"No, I'm sorry, I'm afraid you have the pleasure of making that phone call. Some people prefer to simply mail this handout with an explanatory note," said Dr. Messer.

"Wouldn't he know that he has this? What happens in guys?" asked Meredith.

"Unfortunately, this disease gets spread easily partly because there are no symptoms, especially in men. So, it's entirely possible that Marc has no clue that he has trich or that he gave it to you," answered Dr. Messer.

"Can't you give me a prescription to give to him?" asked Meredith, thinking to herself that there was no way Marc would actually come in to be seen. She didn't honestly care about him, but she did feel sorry for anyone else he had slept with. Well, maybe not for Miss Olive Oyl, but for others.

"No, unfortunately, I cannot legally do that in this state. We have to leave it up to you to tell him, sorry. Do you have any other questions?" Dr. Messer asked.

"When will I have the results of the other tests?"

"Usually they're ready in about three days. You can choose how we notify you when you check out at the front desk. We can have the nurse call you, mail you a letter, or use secure email."

"Do I need a follow-up appointment?" asked Meredith.

"Probably not. Assuming your other tests are all negative, this antibiotic should fix your symptoms for good. Of course, if you have any other concerns, please come back," said the doctor with a smile.

Meredith stood up and gathered her things. With her usual sense of humor beginning to sneak back in, she turned to Dr. Messer and grinned. "You know, the last time I went out with Marc was Halloween. I guess you're 'treating' my 'trich.'"

They shared a laugh, both thinking that next Halloween the phrase "trick or treat" would have a different meaning.

11: Mitch

MITCH PRIED OPEN his eyes and squinted at the clock. 9:52 blinked back at him from his alarm clock, which he had apparently forgotten to set when he crawled in at 3:30 a.m. after studying. "No way," he panicked, leaping out of bed and pulling on his jeans. "I can still make it to my test on time if I run," he rationalized, trying to calm down. Mitch grabbed his backpack and flew out of the dorm. Luckily, the chemistry building was close enough that Mitch slid into his seat in time to hear the final instructions for the test.

"And please, students, everyone pull out your cell phones now and set them on silent," announced the professor.

Dutifully, Mitch fished in his backpack for his phone. As he flipped it open to change the settings to vibrate, he was surprised to see a missed call from his old girlfriend. "I wonder why Jen called," Mitch thought, briefly smiling at the memory of his fiery redheaded ex and her boundless energy.

They had been a great high school couple, but following scholarships to separate universities led to long-distance relationship challenges. Jen broke up with Mitch during Christmas break when she found out Mitch had not stayed faithful. Mitch felt badly that his cheating caused the end of their relationship; however, he maintained that college was the right time to meet other people and casually date around before making a serious commitment. Of course, his definition of this had proven to be quite different than Jen's. Mitch broke the seal to open his test booklet, thoughts of Jen vanishing as he focused on equations and chemical properties.

Mitch dialed Jen as he headed to grab some lunch after the test. After the third ring, as Mitch was assuming he'd have to leave a message, Jen picked up.

"Mitch, I'm going to kill you," Jen whispered fiercely. "Hold on a second while I get to where I can talk."

"And a cheery good morning to you, too, Jen," Mitch countered. "Don't get all pissed at me. I'm returning your call."

"I am pissed at you." hissed Jen. "Hold on a second."

"The nerve of her," Mitch thought, irritated to the core. Out loud, he said, "What can I possibly have done to upset you now? We haven't even seen or talked to each other in four months."

"Okay, I'm outside, now I can talk. Look, I appreciate you calling back. I know I shouldn't have answered the phone like that, but Mitch, I am so furious with you," Jen responded.

"You've clearly established that, but perhaps you'd like to share why you're so upset?" said Mitch in an overly polite tone.

"Yes, I'd love to share, as apparently you did," said Jen, mimicking his tone.

"What are you trying to tell me, Jen?" asked Mitch.

"Mitch, you gave me an STD!" accused Jen.

"Yeah, right," snorted Mitch.

"Mitch, I'm serious. I've been having lots of problems off and on since Christmas, and this morning I found out that it's all from trichomoniasis," explained Jen.

"Trich-a-what?" asked Mitch, still confused.

"Trichomoniasis, Mr. Pre-Med," said Jen angrily. "Put in your language, trich is a single-celled parasite that apparently is the most common nonviral sexually transmitted disease."

"Listen, Jen, I don't know who else you've been with, but I most certainly do not have any disease," retorted Mitch.

"I have not 'been with' anyone except you, dear Mitch. So, unlike you, I don't need to rack my brain to figure out where this came from," spat Jen.

Mitch knew enough about Jen to believe that her statement was true. They were both virgins when they decided to have sex back in high school, and he was definitely the one who had pushed that issue. Mitch would have been surprised and disappointed if Jen had already slept with someone else. Still, the whole idea of him giving her an STD seemed farfetched. He'd only been with a couple of girls. "But, Jen, I don't have any symptoms of anything," he protested.

"My doctor told me that ninety percent of men have no symptoms, so actually, that's not surprising. Not all women get symptoms, but I guess I was lucky," said Jen.

"Did they give you something to treat it?" asked Mitch.

"Yes, so I guess now I'm actually fixed, but I thought you might want to know that you have this disease," said Jen bitterly.

"Well, I'm sorry, but I'm not convinced that I do have it," said Mitch honestly.

"Mitch, let me make this as clear as possible. There is no other way I could have caught trich, except from you. You are the one and only male who has been anywhere near me without wearing clothes. I've only even kissed a few other guys, Mitch. Not from their lack of trying, I might add," she finished.

"I know, I know. It's weird. You can't expect me to feel guilty about something I never even knew that I had," said Mitch defensively.

"Frankly, I don't expect anything from you anymore," retorted Jen. "Let's not prolong this conversation. I'm trying to do the right thing by telling you about the trich. I don't want any other girls to get this disease, regardless of what I may think of your new companions. Please promise me that you will go to the doctor and get treated. I think you owe me that, Mitch."

"Jen, it's not like I'm sleeping around a ton," Mitch started.

"Mitch, honestly, I don't even want to know. Let's not do this to each other. Go to the doctor and get the antibiotics. They're not too much fun to take, but you'll be cured. I've got to get back to class. Good-bye, Mitch," she said definitively.

"Good-bye, and I'm sorry," Mitch replied. This day was not going well.

A few days later, Mitch was sitting in the health center, waiting to see a doctor. After reading everything about trich on the website of the National Institutes of Health, he was convinced that he ought to get treated. Mitch actually hoped to see Jen this summer when they were both home from school, and he knew he wouldn't be able to look her in the eye unless he'd received treatment.

"Mitch Martin?" called out a cute girl holding a chart.

Mitch stood up. "That's me," he said, gathering his backpack and following the girl down the hall.

She chatted as she weighed Mitch and then took his blood pressure and pulse. "Hi, Mitch, I'm Nicole. I'm a medical assistant here at the clinic. Aren't you in the pre-med club? I think I recognize you from the last meeting," she chirped.

"Oh, great," thought Mitch, not the moment I want to be recognized. He did think that Nicole's face looked familiar, with hazel eyes and light brown hair pulled back into a ponytail. Nicole's dark blue scrubs, the uniform of the clinic, took away any other sense of recognition. "I was at that last meeting, but I haven't decided about joining. Everyone seemed pretty intense," said Mitch, trying to shift the focus away from himself.

"Oh, that's because the upperclassmen were all hyped about the MCAT. I think that meeting was right before the last test, and you know if you bomb that admissions test you can kiss your dreams of med school good-bye," Nicole explained. "You really should give it another try before you decide." Nicole finished writing down Mitch's vital signs and then asked, "So, why are you here today?"

Mitch stammered, "I . . . I had some questions for the doctor, that's all. Thanks for getting me all checked in," he smiled convincingly.

"No ongoing complaints, pains, or injuries?" she asked.

"Nope, but thanks," Mitch assured her.

Luckily, Nicole had worked at the clinic long enough to know not to press any further. Mitch sat down in the chair and searched his backpack for some fact sheets that he had printed out from the NIH website. Mitch figured that as a pre-med student, he should at least seem informed. The doctor entered before Mitch made it all the way through his notes.

"Hello, Mitch, I'm Dr. Kwun," she introduced herself as she sat down on her stool and opened his chart. Dr. Kwun was wearing a dark suit under her neatly starched white lab coat. She spoke softly and deliberately. "Looks like you've got some questions for me?"

Mitch set his papers down on his lap. "Yes, I do. To be honest, it's kind of embarrassing."

Dr. Kwun nodded, indicating she was listening.

"I got a phone call from my old girlfriend this week. She has been diagnosed with trichomoniasis, and well, I'm the only person that, um, that..."

"That she's slept with?" Dr. Kwun finished.

"Exactly," said Mitch.

"But, obviously, she's not the only person you've been with," added Dr. Kwun dryly.

"Right," confirmed Mitch.

"And what did you use for protection?" asked Dr. Kwun.

"Jen, my old girlfriend, was on the pill, so we didn't use anything else. I've only been with a couple of other girls, and I used condoms," said Mitch.

"Consistently?" asked Dr. Kwun.

Mitch couldn't read Dr. Kwun at all. Her even tone and fixed expression hid any indication of what she was thinking. "Apparently not," Mitch admitted. He wanted to add that he was not the type of guy who mindlessly sleeps with any girl available, but he felt the need to match Dr. Kwun's somewhat detached manner.

She gestured toward Mitch's papers. "Looks like you've researched trich, so I'll assume you know the basics. Trichomonas is a parasite that is only transmitted from direct genital-to-genital contact. I suppose you're here for treatment and further testing," said Dr. Kwun.

"Further testing?" asked Mitch. "Actually, my impression from reading this stuff was that since the testing is poorly reliable in men, you would automatically treat me."

"For trich, yes, you're absolutely right. Men only test positive around half of the time that they actually have the disease, so we treat all sexual partners of anyone confirmed with trich. I was referring to additional testing to make sure you don't have other sexually transmitted infections as well," Dr. Kwun finished.

"But I don't have any symptoms at all," said Mitch, petulant and now a bit anxious, as he hadn't yet made that leap of logic.

"The majority of STDs are asymptomatic in men, as I'd imagine you found in your research," replied Dr. Kwun. "Please get undressed from the waist down, and sit up here with this drape over your legs. Nicole and I will be back to complete your STD testing in a moment."

"Dr. Kwun, does Nicole have to assist you?" interjected Mitch quickly. "I kind of know her, and it would be really awkward for me."

"If there is another medical assistant available, I'll bring them instead," she responded coolly. "It's our clinic's policy to have a chaperone in the room for any genital exam on males or breast or pelvic exam on women. Please get changed."

Mitch quickly shed his jeans and underwear, following her directions with the drape. "How humiliating can you get?" he wondered, feeling quite vulnerable naked beneath the sheet. Before long, Dr. Kwun returned, followed by a tall, wiry guy wearing dark blue scrubs like the ones Nicole had on.

"This is Sean, he'll be assisting me," said Dr. Kwun, her voice unchanged.

"Thanks," mumbled Mitch.

Sean seemed a bit flustered as he pulled out a whole assortment of tubes and swabs, and set them on the side table tray. Dr. Kwun indicated that Mitch should lie back as she slid out a hidden portion at the end of the exam table, extending the length to accommodate Mitch's legs and feet. She lifted the drape and deftly examined Mitch's genitals, then held out a hand toward Sean. "The blue one, please," she said.

Sean opened a package with blue writing and handed Dr. Kwun what looked like a long, skinny Q-tip. Mitch squeezed his hands into tight fists as she aimed the end of the swab into the tip of his penis. The burning sensation that it caused was bearable, but as Mitch felt a surge of nausea well up, he feared he might pass out.

"That test was for both chlamydia and gonorrhea," Dr. Kwun stated. "I don't see any obvious signs of warts or herpes. We'll draw your blood to test for HIV, syphilis, and hepatitis C."

"So you're finished?" asked Mitch hopefully.

"Yes, except for giving you a prescription to treat your trich," she replied, sliding the leg extender back into the table and helping Mitch to sit up. "Did your ex-girlfriend and/or any of your other sexual partners test positive for anything else?"

"No," he responded, blushing. At the thought of Jen, Mitch was flooded with guilt. Poor Jen, she hadn't done anything to deserve this. He imagined her embarrassment and fury after going through this routine only to be told that she had an STD. She must really hate him, Mitch thought sadly.

"Do you tolerate medicine well?" asked Dr. Kwun as she pulled out her prescription pad.

"What do you mean?" asked Mitch, confused. "I don't often take medicines."

"This particular medicine can cause a metallic taste in your mouth, nausea, abdominal cramping, and/or headaches. We have a choice of giving you a single large dose or seven days of a smaller dose. The single dose has more side effects, but obviously ends more quickly. Also, you can't have any alcohol during treatment, or for three days afterward," Dr. Kwun rattled off.

"I thought it was one extra day without alcohol," said Mitch.

"We recommend three days, in order to be sure it's out of your system. Volunteer to be the designated driver for a week," suggested Dr. Kwun.

"And not to be a pain," Mitch added, "but I read that the extended-release form of the medicine doesn't cause as many side effects. Can I get that?"

"Not from our formulary. We only stock the generic," Dr. Kwun replied evenly. "Which length of treatment would you like?"

Mitch paused. He was beginning to really understand Jen's words when she said the treatment wasn't "too much fun to take." Mitch actually had a very sensitive stomach, at least when it came to new foods or stress. He didn't remember ever taking a medicine that made him feel badly, but then again, he couldn't remember the last time he was even sick. Choosing between a week of possible low-grade symptoms and a couple of days of potentially feeling really crappy was not a great choice. Add in no beer for ten days, with his birthday coming next week, and the decision only got worse.

"Well?" Dr. Kwun asked.

"Um, I guess I'll take the single dose," answered Mitch. "Are they both equally effective?"

"No, they're not. We actually use the seven-day treatment if the single dose fails. However, in our clinic, the single dose works the vast majority of the time," said Dr. Kwun. "Most of the recurrences we see appear to be from partners not getting treated."

"I certainly don't want to take it more than once," Mitch mused, "but I don't want to be sick for a week, either." He couldn't decide.

"Listen, I'm going to write the prescription so you can decide later. The pharmacist will give you fourteen pills. Take one pill twice per day for seven days. Or, if you'd prefer, you can take four pills all at once. Please make certain that you complete a full course, one way or another. Throw away the extra tablets if you take the single dose. Do not give them away, as they can have very dangerous interactions." She tore off the prescription from the pad, and handing it to Mitch, Dr. Kwun concluded, "Here is your lab slip for the blood tests. Your results will be available in three or four days. Check off which way you'd like to be notified down at the bottom. Please send in your other partners to be treated as well. Any questions?"

Mitch shook his head, "No, I think that covers it. Thanks."

Dr. Kwun and Sean left the room, leaving Mitch to get dressed. "Send in your other partners," Dr. Kwun had said, reminding Mitch that he had focused so much on Jen, he hadn't even thought about who gave trich to him in the first place. Mitch had slept with two different girls besides Jen last semester, neither of whom he had spoken to in over six months.

Mitch had no desire to contact either girl. The first, Stacy, didn't even attend school here. Mitch thought she was a relative or friend of his roommate's girlfriend. Stacy had showed up to a dorm party the second week of school. She was older, experienced, willing, and able. Looking back, Mitch couldn't imagine why he had sex with her. "I must have been so surprised to have an open invitation that I acted without thinking," he decided. "I'd lay money down that she's the source of this trich," he thought, mentally kicking himself.

Brooke, the second girl, had been more of a buddy to him. While celebrating after a football game one night, Brooke threw herself at Mitch, pouring out her feelings and trying to convince him she could be a better match with him than Jen. This hookup lasted about a week, until Mitch decided he still had deeper feelings for Jen. Unfortunately, Brooke had hung on, repeatedly called him in tears, begging him to give her another chance. Mitch thought any communication with Brooke could be disastrous. "Then again," Mitch thought, "telling Brooke I likely gave her an STD certainly shouldn't stir up any flames of desire from her."

Mitch finished tying his shoes and slung his backpack over his shoulder. The blood draw at the lab went smoothly, but the pharmacy was packed. He chose not to hang around until the prescription was ready but planned to come back the next day to pick it up. He was still undecided about which treatment to take. "I wonder which one Jen took," Mitch thought. He truly felt awful about giving her an STD and wanted to somehow try to make it up to her. Mitch knew she was too angry with him to talk, but he had to do something. He pulled his cell phone out of his backpack, clicked onto the web, found a number, and dialed.

"Say It with Flowers, this is Debbie, how can I help you?" a female voice answered.

Opening his wallet to grab a credit card, Mitch asked, "Which flowers say, 'I'm really sorry, and I hope you'll forgive me someday'?"

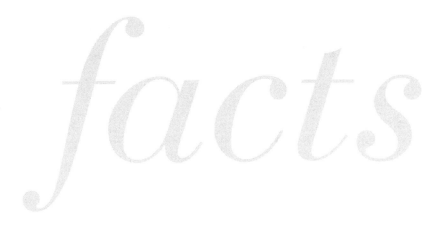

Trichomoniasis Fact Sheet

What is it?

- Trichomoniasis ("trich" for short) is caused by a single-celled protozoan parasite called *Trichomonas vaginalis*.

How common is it?

- The CDC estimates that 7.4 million people are infected in the United States each year.

- Trichomoniasis is thought to be the most common nonviral STD.

How do you get it?

- Trich is transmitted by direct genital-to-genital contact, including, but not limited to, intercourse.

Where on your body do you get it?

- Trich infects the urogenital tract.

- In women, the vagina is the most common location.

- In men, the urethra is the most common site.

How do I know if I have it?

- Many people are asymptomatic.

- Pap smears may identify trich (only 24% sensitivity, meaning that it is detected only 24% of the time that it is actually present).

- Diagnosis is often difficult, because current tests have low sensitivities, ranging from 24 to 83%. This means that nearly half the time disease is present, the tests fail to show a positive result.

What does it look like?

- Normal anatomy.

- Yellow-green or gray discharge in the vagina.

- Redness or small sores on the cervix (seen by the physician during an exam with speculum).

What does it feel like?

- Most men and many women are unaware they have trich.

- 90% of men have no symptoms.

- In the 10% of men with symptoms, most complain of urethral discharge and/or pain with urination or ejaculation.

- Women may have dysparunia (painful intercourse).

- Women can notice a bad odor, itching, and yellow-green, heavy, frothy discharge from the vagina.

How long does it last?

- Trich lasts until it is treated with appropriate antibiotics.

- If symptomatic, it usually manifests between 5 and 28 days from initial contact, but symptoms may come and go, making it difficult to identify a time frame.

Can it be cured?

- Yes, although there is increasing antibiotic resistance to metronidazole.

Can you be re-infected?

- Yes, you can be re-infected.

- Re-infection is common when a partner is not fully treated.

What is the treatment?

- The drug of choice is metronidazole (brand name Flagyl).

- Metronidazole can be given as a single 2 g dose or as a 500 mg tablet taken twice per day for one week.

- Metronidazole has a high incidence of side effects, including primarily nausea, vomiting, headaches, loss of appetite, and metallic taste.

- A person taking metronidazole must abstain from alcohol in all forms during treatment and for 24 hours afterwards.

- The only other drug indicated for trich is tinidazole (brand names Tindamax and Fasigyn), given as a 2 g single dose; no alcohol should be consumed for 72 hours after completion of treatment with this drug.

- If a single-dose treatment fails to eliminate symptoms, and *re-infection is excluded,* then seven days of therapy with metronidazole 500 mg twice per day should be given.

- All sex partners should be treated.

How about alternative therapies?

- Douching is not helpful and likely harmful.

- No herbs or other nonprescription remedies have been proven to eliminate trich.

Are there long-term consequences?

- Trich is associated with giving birth to premature and low-birth-weight infants.

- Trich has been linked with a three- to fivefold increase in transmission or acquisition of HIV.

- Trich is linked with increased risk of infertility and PID (pelvic inflammatory disease).

When are you contagious?

- If you are infected, you are contagious until you are fully treated.

- Latex male condoms can reduce but not eliminate transmission of trich.

How do I avoid getting trich?

- Abstaining from intercourse and from direct genital-to-genital contact will prevent the transmission of trich.

- Using male condoms will decrease but not eliminate the transmission of trich.

- Use new condoms on shared sex toys for each partner, or preferably, do not share sex toys.

If I have trich, how do I avoid giving it to my partner?

- If you have had no prior sexual contact with your partner, abstain from sex and direct genital-to-genital contact until you have completed appropriate antibiotic therapy.

- If you have had prior sexual intimacy with your partner, abstain from sex and from direct genital-to-genital contact until you *both* have completed antibiotic treatment for trich.

Can trich be passed through homosexual contact?

- Since it is not transmitted through oral or anal sex, male-to-male transmission is very unlikely.

- There is evidence of vulva-to-vulva transmission as well as transmission through shared sex toys in women.

Frequently Asked Questions

➤ **Did I catch trich from a toilet seat?**
No, although the parasite has been found on damp towels and underwear, transmission other than by direct genital contact has never been documented.

➤ **Did I get trich from oral or anal sex?**
No, trich cannot survive in the mouth or anus.

➤ **If I just developed symptoms, is it from my current partner?**
Possibly. Women who develop symptoms most often begin to have complaints within 4 to 28 days after exposure, or they may remain asymptomatic for a long period of time.

➤ **If I caught it from my current partner, is he cheating on me?**
Not necessarily. Since men are almost always asymptomatic, they may have been infected for a long time without knowing it.

Additional Information

American College of Obstetricians and Gynecologists
P. O. Box 96920
409 12th Street, SW
Washington, DC 20090-6920
202-863-2518
www.acog.org/publications/patient_education/bp009.cfm

American Social Health Association
P. O. Box 13827
Research Triangle Park, NC 27709
1-800-227-8922
www.ashastd.org/learn/learn_vag_trich.cfm

CDC-INFO
Centers for Disease Control and Prevention
1600 Clifton Road
Atlanta, GA 30333
1-800-CDC-INFO (1-800-232-4636), 1-888-232-6348 TTY
www.cdc.gov/ncidod/dpd/parasites/trichomonas/default.htm

MedlinePlus
National Library of Medicine
8600 Rockville Pike
Bethesda, MD 20894
1-888-FIND-NLM (1-888-346-3656), or 301-594-5983
www.nlm.nih.gov/medlineplus/trichomoniasis.html

PUBIC LICE

12: Zoe

ZOE RELAXED INTO the rhythm of massaging her client's thick blond hair with the rich lather of her favorite shampoo. "You've picked up quite a few natural highlights," she commented.

"You wouldn't believe how hot it was down in Cancun last week," lamented Jason. "I would have melted if the frozen drinks didn't cool me down."

"And this was supposedly work?" said Zoe. "I could have sworn you said you were in Mexico for business."

"Well, entertaining clients is business," Jason defended himself. "That's what the world of sales is all about."

"Tough life," joked Zoe, as she rinsed his hair.

"Yeah, someone's got to do it," Jason flirted back.

Zoe finished towel-drying his hair. "Okay, follow me to my station," she directed.

Jason followed her and sat down in the leather chair, checking out her tight-fitting pants along the way. "Hey look, you match the chair," Jason teased. "Both black leather."

"Yeah, but I sit in cute guys' laps, not the other way around," rebutted Zoe, as she guided Jason into the chair.

This was the fourth time Zoe had cut Jason's hair, and the chemistry between them was simmering. As she leaned forward and brushed off the loose hairs on the cape covering his torso, Zoe was busily trying to think of a subtle way to let him know she was available.

"Hey, Zoe, who are you taking to the after-party tonight?" asked her coworker, Linda, as she walked past Zoe's station.

It was exactly the opening she needed. "Oh, you know me, I'd rather fly solo," Zoe said breezily, gratefully answering in Linda's direction but secretly looking in the mirror for any response from Jason.

"So you don't have a boyfriend right now?" interjected Jason.

Zoe laughed casually. "Nope, too much work. I'm committed to no one. How about you?"

Jason smiled. "I travel too much to get tied down." He stood up, reaching for his wallet. After he stuffed a ten-dollar bill in Zoe's tip jar, Jason turned back to Zoe and handed her his business card. "The bottom number is my cell phone. Why don't you give me a call if you'd like a date to that after-party your friend mentioned?"

"Seriously?" Zoe asked, suddenly nervous.

"Absolutely," reassured Jason. "I have a late meeting 'til roughly eight, but then I'm free. Text me and let me know where to meet you."

"Sounds great," Zoe confirmed happily.

After Jason left, the afternoon passed quickly. Linda and Ty walked over as Zoe was cleaning up her station. "Ah, Jason, the man with the golden hair," teased Linda. "Kind of like that Jason from mythology with the golden fleece, right?"

"Are you comparing him with a sheep?" laughed Zoe. "I'd like to think his mane is far superior to the hair of a barnyard animal."

"And hopefully much cleaner," added Ty, brushing back his purple-streaked hair.

"And less fragrant," finished Linda, holding her nose.

"This conversation has degenerated," announced Zoe. "Come on, Linda, if you're riding with me, let's go."

Before long, Linda and Zoe had transformed themselves into their favorite party outfits, complete with makeup and perfectly styled hair, and were driving over to meet the rest of their friends at Club 21. Zoe had text-messaged Jason where and when to meet up, and she was pleased to see him already at the bar, standing next to Ty and a few of her other coworkers.

"Hey, glad you recognized my friends," said Zoe as she walked up.

"Ty definitely stands out in a crowd," commented Jason, referring to Ty's flamboyant style.

"And, of course, we spotted Golden Boy and called him right over," said Ty, stroking Jason's arm.

"No stealing my date," Zoe directed Ty, stepping in between the two of them and slipping her arm around Jason's waist.

"Don't you know I'd love to, but trust me, I'm not his type," Ty responded with a lewd glance at Jason.

Jason, for his part, looked very uncomfortable. "Yeah, I prefer ...blonds," he said with a weak smile. "Seriously, I'm glad you're here, Zoe. I'm usually up for the club scene, but after being stuck in meetings all day, this pounding music and the flashing lights are a bit overstimulating. How about you and I sneak out and head down the street to my favorite bistro for some strawberries and chocolate fondue?"

"I never refuse chocolate," said Zoe. "I'm game."

"No fair, chocolate and Golden Boy," whined Linda discreetly as Zoe handed over the car keys. "See you tomorrow."

"Gee, was it something I said?" Ty bantered.

The next day at work, everyone was grilling Zoe.

"How was your date?" asked Debra, the haircolorist.

"I'll bet he was as yummy as he looks," offered Ty.

"More importantly, does he have any friends?" asked Linda.

"Really, guys, back off. Jason is cute enough, but I think he's too conservative for me," Zoe answered. "I think he was a bit put off by our crowd. Maybe he's more mature than us, I don't know. I will say that he was right about the bistro, though. Jason ordered some amazing wine to go along with our chocolate dessert. That part was heavenly."

"So did you sleep with him?" persisted Ty, ever the gossip.

"Technically, yes, I slept with him, meaning we shared the same bed, which, by the way, was immaculately made up, matching the rest of his perfect apartment. But no, I did not have sex with him, not that it's any of your business," added Zoe. "To be honest, I'm not that into him. He's all about *Newsweek* and stock futures, and frankly I'm more about enjoying the here and now for a few more years."

"So are you going out with him again?" asked Debra.

Zoe shook her head. "I don't think so. Not unless I need a date to a family function. He's the kind of guy they'd think was perfect for me."

Two nights later, lying in bed, the image of Jason in his bed was foremost in Zoe's mind as she found herself repeatedly scratching her pubic area. "This itch is driving me nuts," thought Zoe, "it's worse than last night." She vaguely remembered Jason scratching his crotch during the night but had written it off to a rude male habit. "Maybe I'm imagining the worst, but I've got to get this checked out. I'm going to claw myself to death."

The next morning, Zoe was able to get an early walk-in appointment with her family doctor. Dr. Patel was always full of energy and meticulously dressed. Zoe was not her stylist, but she appreciated Dr. Patel's chin-length bobbed cut that worked well with her thick dark hair.

"Hi, Zoe," greeted Dr. Patel as she entered the exam room. "What brings you in today?"

"Hi, Dr. Patel. Nice haircut, by the way," Zoe complimented. "It's kind of embarrassing, but I'm here because I've got an unbelievably itchy crotch."

"Is there a rash?" asked the doctor.

"I didn't see one," answered Zoe.

"How long has it been there?"

"Just the last few days," replied Zoe.

"Are you using new laundry detergent? Or any new soaps, gels, lotions, or shampoos?" quizzed Dr. Patel.

"I did get a new bath gel last week," mused Zoe.

"But the only spot you're itching is your groin?" verified the physician.

"Well, sometimes I'm itching all over, but I think that's in my head. The only part that is driving me nuts is my crotch," said Zoe.

"Any vaginal discharge or burning when you pee?"

"None," assured Zoe.

"Any new sexual partners?" Dr. Patel inquired.

"Not really, but I slept in someone's bed this week," admitted Zoe.

"Okay, then let's take a look," said Dr. Patel. Zoe was already dressed in a patient gown, without underwear as the nurse had instructed. She lay back for the doctor to examine her.

"I can see where you've been scratching," commented the doctor as she looked at Zoe. Dr. Patel pulled over a large magnifying glass with a built-in lamp that looked exactly like the one Zoe's mom used when she did needlepoint. "This helps my rapidly aging eyes," she joked as she continued her exam. "Oh, here's the problem," she declared. "Zoe, brace yourself, because you're not going to like this. It looks like you've got pubic lice. I'm going to go look at one of your hairs under the microscope, but I believe these are nits."

Zoe recoiled. "Gross," she proclaimed. "If there is one thing hair stylists can't stand, it's lice. Oh man, I'm definitely going to itch everywhere now."

"I'll be right back," said Dr. Patel, leaving the room carrying the hair in her gloved hands.

Zoe sat up and looked through the magnifying lens that was still suspended over her crotch. She did not need the doctor's confirmation to know that indeed, her pubic hair had multiple nits. Zoe recoiled in disgust as she started picking at and removing the nits with her fingernails.

Dr. Patel returned to find Zoe busily extracting nits. "Sorry, Zoe, but as apparently you can see, it's definitely pubic lice nits, better known as crabs."

"Dr. Patel, our worst nightmare at the salon is one of our clients bringing in their daughter with a thick head of hair all full of lice, asking us to give them the cutest, shortest haircut possible. We call them 'pediculosis princesses.' It happens every month or two, and we all walk around scratching our heads for a week afterwards," shuddered Zoe.

"I understand," said the doctor. "At least this is a much smaller area to cover," she said optimistically.

"But way more disgusting," disagreed Zoe. "You know, I washed this guy's hair before our date. He was actually my client," she explained. "I can assure you that he didn't have any lice on his head. Isn't it the same bug?"

"No, actually, it's not. Pubic lice strongly prefer the coarse pubic hair, and only branch out to axillary hair, eyelashes, or beards, and mustaches," instructed the doctor.

"Axillary?" questioned Zoe.

"Armpits."

Zoe quickly crossed her arms as though to protect her armpits from invasion, a look of revulsion on her face. "Yuck. I think I know where I got mine, but where do most people get them? This guy's hygiene seemed excellent, and his house was unbelievably clean. I'm sure he must have a maid. He is the last person I would suspect to have lice."

"Does he travel?" asked the doctor.

"Yes, he says that he travels a ton for his job. He just got back from Mexico," said Zoe.

"Perhaps he got it from hotel linens that were infected and not adequately cleaned," said Dr. Patel.

Zoe shrugged. "All I really want to know at this point is how do I get rid of them?"

"Well, there are several over-the-counter products to choose from," said Dr. Patel. "We generally don't use the prescription medicine, Lindane, unless the other products don't work, because it has more side effects."

"I want the strongest one that works the best," pleaded Zoe. "Please go ahead and give me the prescription one. I don't want these nasty little crabs one minute longer than I absolutely have to deal with them."

"Truly, you're not pregnant, nursing, or too young, and you don't have any open sores, so there shouldn't be any problem with that," Dr. Patel reasoned out loud, reaching for her prescription pad. She wrote out the script and handed it to Zoe.

"Really, I'd recommend the over-the-counter products. If for some reason they don't work, then fill this prescription. Follow the directions exactly. More is not better in this case. You only leave the shampoo on for four minutes, then rinse it off thoroughly. Finish picking off the nits after you shampoo. The most important part is treating all your linens as well. Wash your towels, sheets, blankets, and clothes in hot soapy water, and then dry them in a dryer for at least twenty minutes. If you have anything in those categories that can't be washed and dried, bag them up in Ziploc or sealed bags and leave them there for fourteen days."

"No way, I'm throwing everything out," professed Zoe. "I've been looking for an excuse to get new bedding, and this is it."

"I wouldn't get new stuff until you're sure you are completely treated," cautioned the doctor. "Some people need a second treatment a week or so later. The medicine only kills the adult form of the lice. If any eggs are missed when you manually remove the nits, they will hatch in about a week and restart the cycle."

"How long do they live?" asked Zoe.

"Eggs—the nits—last roughly seven days, then nymphs, which are immature adults, crawl out. It takes another week for the nymphs to become adult lice capable of laying eggs. An adult female lays up to ten eggs per day and lives roughly two weeks. Adult lice can only survive one to two days off a human, though."

"What about my couch or other chairs?" asked Zoe.

"Assuming you've only sat on your couch in clothes, it's not a problem. If you slept on it in just underwear, I'd spray it with the over-the-counter anti-lice sprays," answered the doctor.

"When will I stop itching?"

"The itch often stays for several days after you've completed treatment. Don't worry about it unless you continue to see nits. Sometimes putting calamine lotion on the itchy spots will help, or taking an oral antihistamine like diphenhydramine, which is Benadryl, at bedtime will help calm down the itch and let you sleep easier." Dr. Patel paused, then finished, "Remember to let your friend from the other night know, so he can get treated, too."

"You can be sure I'll let him know," smiled Zoe sarcastically. As she got dressed, her friends' barnyard jokes popped back into her head. "Maybe he does belong on a farm," Zoe smirked to herself. She could only imagine the new nicknames Jason would have at the salon. Golden Boy would be out, replaced with Pediculosis Prince, Lice Lord, Crab Crotch, or worse. Good thing she wasn't hooked on him. Heaven help him if he ever returned for a haircut. She flipped open her cell phone and scrolled to find his number from the other day.

"Jason," she text-messaged, "you brought back more than a tan and highlights from Mexico. Call me."

13: Ryan

"PROMISE ME THAT YOU won't do anything stupid just to impress all your buddies," Elise begged. "I know how you all try to out-macho one another, especially after a few beers," she added.

Ryan smirked and rolled his eyes, glad that his fiancée wasn't able to see his expression as he spoke into his cell phone. "Really, everything will be fine. Don't get so worked up. It's more about a guys' weekend hanging out at the lake than the bachelor party," he said.

"Look, you know I'm not the typical hysterical bride," Elise replied calmly, "but I can picture Nick or Joe getting you all to jump in the lake for a midnight swim or something after you've been drinking all night, and I don't want you to drown or break an arm."

"Ah, don't worry, the strippers will be here by midnight, so no one will want to leave the house," Ryan joked, as the passengers in his car erupted in laughter.

"Okay, now you're pushing your luck. You know I trust you, Ryan, but your high school friends are another deal," Elise warned.

"I'm teasing, Elise. Go enjoy your girls' spa weekend and relax with all the pampering your heart desires. I promise to keep the guys under control, or if I can't do that, I at least promise to lock myself in a room away from them," Ryan laughed.

"Fair enough," sighed Elise. "Have fun and be safe. I love you."

"Love you, too," responded Ryan quickly in a low voice, snapping his flip phone shut to end the call.

A falsetto chorus of "We love you, too" echoed throughout the car, as Ryan's groomsmen took up the chant. Who knew what this weekend would bring?

The caravan pulled up to Nick's lake house, and guys poured out of the cars. "Ah, the famous 'love shack' of the not-so-famous Nick," announced Rob as they grabbed their bags and headed into the house.

"Trust me, it's famous to the women I've brought up here," bragged Nick.

"As long as it's got plenty of beer and food, that's all I care about," interjected Zach.

"Don't worry, Barbie and I drove up last weekend, and we stocked the place to the hilt," assured Nick. "We've got enough food and drinks for an army."

"But is that enough for Ryan's last weekend as a free man?" asked Cory. "And who is Barbie? Is that really her name?"

"Barbie is my date for the wedding, and yes, no kidding, it's her name. Anyway, if the food runs out, that's what pizza delivery is for," said Nick, "and there's a liquor store only fifteen minutes away."

The gang swarmed into the house, most of them dumping their bags in the living room and heading out to the deck to pop open a beer and check out the lake. Ryan headed to the back of the house and staked claim on a bedroom so he wouldn't have to sleep on the floor or the couch, as both had clearly seen better days. "The ultimate bachelor pad for my bachelor party," thought Ryan, looking around the room. The bed was unmade, with sheets and blankets tossed open from the previous occupant. "It must be time for me to get married, when this actually looks unappealing to me," decided Ryan. He tossed his stuff on the bed and went to join his friends.

The long weekend exceeded Ryan's expectations. Everyone got along fine, with only a few exceptions that Ryan wrote off to irritable attitudes from morning hangovers. The guys cruised the lake on Nick's boat and jet skis, drinking, eating, and repeating old stories of their high school glory days, their accomplishments embellished more with every telling. True to form, Nick brought in a few strippers Saturday night, but Ryan wasn't even tempted to stray. He enjoyed hanging out with his old buddies, but now that the weekend was over, more than anything Ryan was looking forward to his honeymoon the next week.

Elise and Ryan had splurged on an amazing trip to the Virgin Islands, where they planned to scuba dive, sail, relax, and escape from the craziness of their overblown wedding. "Why is it that weddings always seem to take on a life of their own?" thought Ryan. Through family friends and relatives, their guest list had doubled from their original plan. Ryan realized, though, that Elise had much more on her plate as the bride than he had to deal with as the groom. "Oh well, all I've got left to do these last two days is get all the guys to do the final fitting for the tuxedos and figure out a schedule to pick up friends and relatives from the airport."

Ryan shifted uncomfortably in his car seat as he headed across town toward the tuxedo rental store. He realized he'd been scratching at his crotch off and on for the last day or so, although it wasn't bothering him now nearly as much as it did during the night. The night before, Ryan had woken up multiple times clawing at his pubic area from an intense itch, but when the irritation faded in the morning, Ryan had completely forgotten about it. He reached under the seatbelt for a better angle to scratch. Now that he was conscious of it again, Ryan was worried. "I hope I'm not getting poison ivy again," he fretted.

The summer before, Ryan had had such a bad case of poison ivy that the rash and itch came and went for almost six weeks. He had required two separate rounds of steroid pill packs and one shot of additional steroids. They had not initially realized that his roommate's dog Corby was the source, constantly reexposing him. Ryan learned that the irritants from poison ivy stay on animal fur, and once they quit letting Corby run through the bushes at the park, Ryan's rash finally stayed clear.

At any rate, the last thing Ryan wanted to deal with during his honeymoon was an itchy rash in his groin that he knew would only get worse with sun exposure and heat. Ryan spotted an urgent care clinic and pulled into the parking lot, thinking he could pop in, get a quick steroid shot, and avoid a severe reaction. Looking at his watch, Ryan felt that he had plenty of time before he needed to be at the rental store. Ryan considered calling his regular doctor back home, but even if Dr. Kubiak agreed to call in some medicine, Ryan felt like he would respond more quickly if he could get an injection. He entered the clinic and checked in.

Before long, Ryan was following a young lady down the hallway, where she weighed him and chatted pleasantly while taking his vital signs and guiding him into an exam room. "I'm Susan, Dr. Kent's medical assistant," she noted. "What seems to be bothering you today?"

"Well, I was at the lake last weekend, and I think perhaps I'm getting poison ivy," explained Ryan. "I'm actually getting married this weekend…"

"Congratulations," Susan chirped.

"Thanks. Anyway, we're headed to the Virgin Islands…"

"Lucky dogs," she interjected.

"Uh, yeah. But, I don't want to head down there with poison ivy," Ryan finished quickly. "Do you think I can get a steroid shot?"

"I don't see why not," Susan answered. "We give them all the time for poison ivy, and we've been seeing a bunch of it lately. We'll see what Dr. Kent says in a few minutes when he comes in. Where is your rash?"

"In my crotch, I guess. To be honest, I haven't even looked to see if there's a rash. It feels pretty much like when I had poison ivy last year, though. I don't live in town anymore, so when I saw your clinic, I thought it would be best to come in and treat this as soon as possible."

"Fair enough," Susan agreed. "Why don't you change into this gown, with your underwear off, please, so Dr. Kent can examine you and get you all fixed up for your wedding."

"Okay," said Ryan, reaching for the gown. Once Susan left, Ryan undressed and put on the gown, hoping he had guessed correctly by having it open to the back, like a hospital gown. He looked at his groin and saw only one bright red, raised line toward the edge of his pubic hair. "Good," he thought, "it doesn't look too bad yet." The rash last year had covered his groin, belly, back, and thighs, plus he had a few marks on his forearms. Ryan sat on the end of the exam table, grabbing a magazine from a basket on the floor to kill the time while he waited. Considering how quickly he had been taken back into a room, it was a long wait for the doctor to arrive. Ryan had read two *People* magazines and was halfway through a *Reader's Digest* when an older gentleman wearing cowboy boots, jeans, a button-down shirt, and a full-length white lab coat entered the room.

"Howdy, I'm Dr. Kent," said the man, extending his hand.

Ryan returned his firm handshake. "Hi, I'm Ryan. Thanks for seeing me."

"Sorry about the wait, we had a few emergencies slip in before you," apologized Dr. Kent.

"If you can fix me by Saturday, it's all good," responded Ryan.

"Oh that's right," said the doctor. "Susan mentioned you're getting married this weekend. Congratulations. I'll do my best to solve your problem by then, but no promises till I see what we're dealing with."

"I think it's poison ivy. It doesn't look that bad yet, but I had a terrible case last year," explained Ryan. "It itches really bad."

"When did you first notice it bothering you?" asked the doctor.

"I think it started yesterday. It definitely was itching last night, and all day today."

"And do you know where you might have been exposed?" inquired Dr. Kent.

"My bachelor party was out at the lake last weekend. We hiked through a bunch of weeds when we walked out to my friend's dock, so it could have been there," answered Ryan.

"Bachelor party, eh? Any new sexual partners?" said Dr. Kent.

"No way," replied Ryan, somewhat offended. "Why do you ask?"

"Well, you know what they say, son. If a dog itches, sometimes it's ticks, and sometimes it's fleas."

"What? I'm not following you," puzzled Ryan.

"I simply mean that you could have poison ivy, and you could have caught something else," clarified the doctor. "You would not be the first groom to catch something that made his groin itch from his bachelor party," he chuckled.

"Yeah, but I would be the last. My fiancée would kill me," Ryan tried to joke back. "But seriously, it's not a concern."

"All right, then let's take a look. Go ahead and lay back, son," instructed Dr. Kent, grabbing a pair of gloves out of a box and slipping them on his hands.

Ryan wondered what the doctor was doing when Dr. Kent grabbed the otoscope off the wall. "Isn't that to look in ears?" Ryan asked.

"Yes, but it's also a great lighted magnifying glass," clarified the doctor.

Dr. Kent lifted Ryan's patient gown, and quickly focused in on the red streak Ryan had noticed earlier. "This is an irritated scratch right here, but there are no blisters or clear discharge or anything suggestive of poison ivy," commented Dr. Kent. He continued to look around Ryan's thighs and pubic region until something else caught his attention. "Bingo," he exclaimed.

"What?" asked Ryan, rising up to his elbows.

"Unfortunately, son, you have indeed picked up a crawling critter, but not ticks or fleas," Dr. Kent declared. "You've got crabs."

"Crabs? No way. I told you, I didn't sleep with anybody, I swear it," Ryan argued defensively.

"Where did you sleep last weekend?" inquired the doctor.

Ryan closed his eyes and let his head drop forward, shaking it back and forth. "In my friend's disgusting bachelor pad," he admitted.

"I'm guessing the sheets were less than clean, then," responded Dr. Kent.

"Apparently," confirmed Ryan.

"Well, the good news is that it's not poison ivy, so you don't need steroids. The bad news is that this is extremely contagious. You've got to be sure that you and all of your clothing and bedding are completely treated, so you don't give this to your bride this weekend. That most certainly would not be a welcome wedding gift," concluded Dr. Kent.

"Will it be gone by this weekend?" asked Ryan nervously.

"Well, the medicine kills off any adult lice, but if you don't remove all of the eggs, which are called nits, then they could hatch next week on your honeymoon."

"How do I get rid of the eggs?"

"You can use a fine-toothed comb. They usually sell special combs along with the medicated shampoos that kill the lice," responded Dr. Kent.

"And you said I need to treat my clothes and bedding, too? What do I have to do for that?" inquired Ryan.

"Everything that can be washed in the washing machine should be washed in hot water with detergent and then dried in the dryer for at least twenty minutes. Anything that can't be washed needs to be put in an airtight bag and sealed off for ten to fourteen days. There are also medicated sprays that you can spray on couches and chairs," explained the doctor.

Ryan was going through everything in his head, realizing he would have to make time to wash all of his clothes that were back at the hotel. Add in a trip to a laundromat to his to-do list. Suddenly, it seemed the clock was ticking too fast, with extra tasks cropping up left and right. "Okay, so where do I get the medicine? Is it prescription?" he asked.

"No, there are a couple brands that you can buy straight over the counter," replied Dr. Kent. "We generally don't use the prescription type unless the other ones don't seem to work, because the prescription one has more potential side effects. My nurse will give you a handout with the names of all the available products, as well as printed instructions for treating your clothes and bedding. You should be able to pick up everything across the street at the local pharmacy or grocery store. If I were you, I'd pick up a second treatment to take with you on your honeymoon just in case anything else crops up, although usually one application will take care of it. Any other questions?" asked Dr. Kent.

"I don't think so," said Ryan thoughtfully. "I really need to get rid of these, uh, crabs as fast as possible. My fiancée will be pretty freaked out when she finds out about this problem. Luckily, we've barely seen each other this week."

"Have you shared a bed, or any other spot, since your party?" asked the doctor.

"No, we haven't," Ryan answered happily.

"Great, then she shouldn't have been exposed. My best wishes to the bride," smiled Dr. Kent, "and good luck to you."

Ryan got dressed, paid the bill at the front desk and double checked that he had the treatment instructions as he got into his car. He started the car and checked his watch, trying to decide if he had time to head into the pharmacy across the street before he headed to the tuxedo rental store.

"Oh man," Ryan suddenly agonized, "what are we going to do about the tuxedos?" With everyone at the same house last weekend, it was certainly conceivable that Ryan was not the only one that had acquired crabs. And now, they were all supposed to go and try on rental tuxedos. Didn't the doctor tell him that crabs could be spread through clothing? Gross. Ryan didn't want to be responsible for spreading this disease around. They would simply all have to get treated before they could go to the tuxedo shop. "Man, they are never ever going to let me live this down," Ryan thought.

He dialed information on his cell phone, and soon was connected with the shop. "Hi, this is Ryan..."

"Ryan Anderson?" asked the salesman at the store.

"Yes, that's me," replied Ryan.

"Great. Two of your groomsmen have arrived here ahead of you, and we can get started on their measurements, but we'll obviously need you here for your final fitting, as well. Are you far away?" asked the man.

"Actually, uh, something's come up. I...I can't make it there today," stammered Ryan. "Will it be a problem if we all show up first thing tomorrow?"

"Well," snipped the salesman with some irritation, "I can't promise we'll still have everything, but we'll make do. Can you be here promptly at ten in the morning when we open?"

Ryan breathed a sigh of relief. "Yes, ten is no problem. Thank you. Can you ask my friends to call me on my cell phone?"

"So you can tell them what 'came up'?" jibed the clerk.

"Yeah. Sorry again," said Ryan, as he ended the call.

Within seconds, his phone was ringing. "Ryan?" said Nick, "What's up? I thought Elise said we had to get this done today. You know, she's going to blame me if we don't get the right penguin suits."

Ryan practically bit his tongue. "Oh, Elise is going to blame you, all right," he retorted. "Nick, do me a favor and call me back from outside the rental shop. I don't want you to repeat what I'm going to tell you out loud."

"What are you talking about? The guy says he can take our measurements while we're here," Nick responded.

"Seriously, please tell him you'll be back in the morning. Come on, Nick, don't mess around. Step outside and call me right back," Ryan said, hanging up.

Again, the phone rang almost immediately. "Okay, okay, I'm outside, but Ben is still in there. What is so important?" Nick asked impatiently.

"Nick, I got crabs from your love shack last weekend," accused Ryan.

"Crabs? Isn't that pubic lice? Are you kidding me? I think you're being paranoid," Nick assessed.

"Trust me, I walked out of the doctor's office a minute ago. The guy found crab eggs in my crotch," rebutted Ryan.

"There's no way, Ryan. How could you get that from my lake house? If you did, it was from those strippers. Dude, I thought you stayed pretty much out of their way," said Nick, laughing through the phone.

"Nick, it's not funny. I got them from the sheets, and you slept there the weekend before, so I'd bet you have them, too. For that matter, I think we probably all need to get treated before we go put on rental suits and spread this around even more. Meet me at my hotel, and I'll pick up the medicine for everyone at the pharmacy."

"Okay, Mr. Responsible, but I think you're going overboard," replied Nick.

"By the way, I'd rather that Elise and the other women not know about this," Ryan suggested.

"So they won't get crabby?" teased Nick.

Ryan rolled his eyes. With these guys, he'd be lucky if this didn't become the main theme of the weekend. How would his in-laws-to-be react if they found out? What a hassle. "Whatever, Nick. Go ahead, get it out of your system, and make all the jokes you want with me today. I'm seriously asking you, as my best man, to help me put this to rest so it doesn't ruin the wedding weekend for Elise. See you at the hotel, okay?"

"Gotcha," Nick chuckled, and true to his nature, couldn't resist adding, "We'll bug out of here right now. Don't worry, I'll think of an excuse that's not too...lousy."

Ryan shook his head, but he had to laugh at the bad pun. Nick's quick wit had earned him the reputation as the class clown growing up, always keeping the gang laughing. Ryan hoped he could convince Nick to resist the temptation to talk about crabs during his best-man toast at the rehearsal dinner.

facts

Pubic Lice Fact Sheet

What is it?

- "Crabs" is the common name for pubic lice. The scientific name for this tiny, 1.2 mm adult six-legged parasitic insect is *Phthirus pubis*.

- Another medical name for infestation is pediculosis.

How common is it?

- Pubic lice infestation is common worldwide.

- The National Institute of Allergy and Infectious Disease estimates 3 million new people are infected in the United States each year.

- The incidence rate of pubic lice is 1 in 90 people in the United States.

How do you get it?

- Crabs are transmitted most often through intercourse but also by direct contact with infected bed linens, clothing, or towels.

- People trying on bathing suits at stores without wearing underwear can transmit or pick up pubic lice.

Where on your body do you get it?

- Pubic lice primarily infest pubic hair.

- They can also infest armpit hair, eyebrows, and eyelashes.

How do I know if I have it?

- Pubic lice cause moderate to severe itching, which is typically worse at night.

- Close inspection of pubic hair reveals small white or yellow oval dots, usually fixed near the base of the hair shaft. These are nits, the eggs of the lice.

- Adult lice can often be found in seams of clothing.

What does it look like?

- The creature itself has a round body with six legs. The front two legs are larger, closely resembling the pincer claws of a crab when looked at under magnification. Adults are tan to grayish-white.

- Small white dots on the pubic hairs can be seen with the naked eye.

- Because the itching leads to scratching, most people have scratch marks, called excoriations, around the pubic region.

- Sometimes the bites will cause a bluish-gray reaction in the skin.

- Scratching and breaking open the skin can cause secondary bacterial infections, which are called impetigo.

What does it feel like?

- Pubic lice need human blood to survive, so they bury their heads in the pubic hair follicle, excreting an irritating substance into the skin that causes moderate to severe itching.

How long does it last?

- Pubic lice last until the person is treated with appropriate medicine and environmental infestation is eliminated (to avoid re-infestation).

- Each female adult louse lays 30 to 50 eggs during her life span.

- If an infestation is with many adults, symptoms can begin immediately.

- If an infestation is only a few adults, symptoms may not be obvious for 2 to 4 weeks as the adults lay eggs, and the eggs take over a week to hatch, mature, and proliferate.

Can it be cured?

- Yes, but the environment must be treated as well to prevent re-infestation.

Can you be re-infected?

- Yes, you can be re-infected.

What is the treatment?

- Over-the-counter medicines are available, containing permethrin or permethrin with piperonyl butoxide, both agents that kill only adult lice.

- Prescription washes contain hexachlorocyclohexane, brand name Lindane, another adult pediculocide, which must be used with caution due to potential nervous system side effects. Only a physician or other authorized prescribing medical personnel should decide whether or not this is the correct treatment for your lice.

- Over-the-counter medicated shampoos are applied to dry pubic hair, worked in for 5 to 10 minutes, and thoroughly rinsed. Remaining nits should then be removed with a fine-toothed comb.

- Usually a single treatment is all that is needed, but some infestations require a second treatment 5 to 10 days later (to remove the nymph and adult stages of lice that may have hatched from any remaining nits).

- For eyelash or eyelid infestations, only petroleum jelly can be used. No shampoo, cream, or ointment containing anti-lice medications should ever be used on the eyes.

- Bedding and clothing must be washed in hot water and dried in a hot dryer for at least 20 minutes.

- Items that cannot be washed can be sprayed with a medicated spray or must be sealed in plastic bags for 10 to 14 days to suffocate the lice.

- All intimate contacts, including not only sexual partners, but anyone who has shared bedding, linens or clothing, and their environments should be treated at the same time.

How about alternative therapies?

- Occlusive dressings such as petroleum jellies or mayonnaise have limited effectiveness and are not recommended.

- Shaving is not necessary to treat lice infestation and does not prevent infection.

Are there long-term consequences?

- Lice infestation by itself does not lead to long-term problems.

- Secondary infections from repeated scratching could rarely cause further complications or scarring.

When are you contagious?

- If you are infected, you are contagious until you and your environment are fully treated.

- Pubic lice are thought to be potentially the most infectious sexually transmitted disease.

- One contact with an infected partner results in a 95% chance of transmission.

- Condoms do not reduce transmission of pubic lice, because they do not cover pubic hair.

Can crabs be transmitted between homosexual partners?

- Absolutely.

How do I avoid catching crabs?

- Abstain from intercourse and direct genital contact with new partners (and their bedding).

- Wear underwear when trying on swimsuits or undergarments in stores.

If I have crabs, how do I avoid giving it to my partner?

- Meticulously follow the medication instructions to rid your body, your clothing, and your linens of the pubic lice, and do not have intimate contact for 10 days after initial treatment.

- If you have been intimate with any partners during your infestation, they need to treat themselves and their environment as well, to avoid passing the lice back and forth.

Frequently Asked Questions

➤ Do you have to have sex to catch crabs?
No. Pubic lice can be transmitted from close genital contact or through infested bed linens, clothing, or towels.

➤ Did I catch crabs from a toilet seat?
Very unlikely. Pubic lice don't live long off humans and don't have the capacity to grip onto smooth surfaces such as a toilet seat.

➤ Did I get crabs from oral sex?
Unlikely. Potentially, you could get pubic lice infestation on your eyelashes or facial hair from performing oral sex.

➤ Are pubic lice the same as head lice?
No. Pubic lice are not found on the scalp. They can be distinguished under the microscope by their body type: pubic lice are short and round, whereas head lice are longer and oval shaped. Treatment, however, is similar.

➤ Did I catch this from trying on swimsuits?
Possibly. Always wear underwear when trying on swimsuits or undergarments to decrease (although not eliminate) chances of getting this infestation.

➤ Did I get this from my dog or cat?

No. Pubic lice cannot live on or be transmitted by animals, only humans.

Additional Information

American Social Health Association
P. O. Box 13827
Research Triangle Park, NC 27709
1-800-227-8922
www.ashastd.org/learn/learn_crabs.cfm

CDC-INFO
Centers for Disease Control and Prevention
1600 Clifton Road
Atlanta, GA 30333
1-800-CDC-INFO (1-800-232-4636), 1-888-232-6348 TTY
www.cdc.gov/ncidod/dpd/parasites/lice/factsht_pubic_lice.htm

MedlinePlus
National Library of Medicine
8600 Rockville Pike
Bethesda, MD 20894
1-888-FIND-NLM (1-888-346-3656), or 301-594-5983
www.nlm.nih.gov/medlineplus/ency/article/000841.htm

14: Evan

EVAN WALKED IN THE door from work, exhausted from standing on his feet all afternoon. For Christmas break, he had returned to his old summer job as a grocery checker. Being back at home was a mixed blessing. Evan hated having to follow someone else's schedule, but it was wonderful to come home to delicious home-cooked meals instead of the slop that passed for food back at the college cafeteria. Tonight he smelled his favorite—good old spaghetti and meatballs.

"Oh good, you're back in time for dinner. We were sitting down to eat. Come join us after you wash your hands," his mom said.

Evan managed to wash his hands without any smart-aleck comments about being old enough to know how to do this without his mother's advice and sat down to eat. He would be headed back to school and those fast food dinners in a few days, so he knew he'd better savor this meal.

"By the way, the doctor's office called us today saying they couldn't reach you on your cell phone, and Dr. Litz wants you to come in tomorrow to discuss your lab work from your physical this week. I made an appointment for you at eight fifteen tomorrow morning, so it won't interfere with your work schedule. I hope everything's okay." The last comment was more of a question than a statement. Evan shrugged as he grabbed some butter to slather on his second roll.

"I'm sure it's no big deal, Mom. Didn't they have anything later in the morning? Hanna and I are going out to a late movie tonight."

"You're headed back out?"

"Don't even go there, honey," Evan's dad said to his mom, placing his hand on her arm. "Take a cab if you guys have anything to drink, son."

Evan rolled his eyes, saying, "Dad, you know I'm underage anyway. We're going to a movie, not bar hopping on Sixth Street." The rest of the meal was fairly quiet, with Evan finishing off a third plate of spaghetti and meatballs while his mom discreetly tried to pump him for information about his new girlfriend.

His parents had been furious last semester when they realized his first girlfriend in college—actually, his first serious girlfriend ever— was not only six years older than him but had already been married and divorced. Evan had never been particularly impressed with girls his age in high school. They were always obsessed with superficial things like fashion, reality television shows, and gossip. Courtney had been the first girl who ever shared his passions about more important things, like social justice, and also happened to share his taste in music. She had asked him out to hear a local band after work one night, and he had quickly fallen for her head over heels. When Evan later found out that she was still involved sporadically with her ex-husband, he was heartbroken. He stayed with Courtney for a couple of months but finally broke up with her when he realized that she seemed incapable of making a clean break from her ex.

At any rate, there was no threat of any unfinished business with his new girlfriend, Hanna. She was actually one year younger than Evan, still in high school, and was a virgin when they began dating a few weeks ago. Evan had really enjoyed the sexual intimacy that Courtney had taught him, and he quickly became sexually active with Hanna. Hanna was already on the pill to control her painful periods, but Evan made sure to use condoms to protect against disease as well. He knew he should have been more consistent about using condoms with Courtney, but he was going to be sure that he and Hanna would be completely safe.

The next morning, his alarm clock went off much too early. He grabbed a clean t-shirt and jeans from his laundry basket; his mom must have washed his clothes for him the night before. As he drove over to Dr. Litz's office, Evan began to wonder what was so important that she wanted to bring him in to discuss his bloodwork. He had had his annual physical with her a couple of days earlier in the week. He had agreed to STD testing after admitting that he had not always been perfect about wearing a condom. Could it be gonorrhea or something? He had absolutely no symptoms. Maybe his blood count was low again. A couple of years ago he had been vegetarian for a year and had become a little anemic. He laughed at that when he thought about how much he had enjoyed Mom's meatballs. Not much chance of that this year.

Evan checked in with the receptionist, showed them his insurance card for the second time in three days, and forked over his ten-dollar co-pay. He went through the motions of being weighed and getting his temperature and blood pressure taken, practically falling asleep while he sat in the chair waiting for the doctor to come in. Dr. Litz actually came in pretty quickly, but she didn't seem to be her usual joking self. Evan sat up, his heart suddenly racing. "Okay, what's up?" he asked.

"Evan, I've known you since you were a little boy. You know that I always tell you the truth. Well, now I've got some news, and it's scary, but I'm going to tell you everything, and we'll get through it, okay?" Dr. Litz was looking him straight in the eye and had put her hand on his knee as she pulled her rolling stool right in front of him. Evan was wide awake now and felt vaguely nauseated as his heart pounded practically out of his chest.

"What, what is it?" he demanded.

"You know we tested you for all the usual bloodwork plus STDs. Well, everything else came back normal, but your HIV test came back positive."

"HIV? Oh my God, HIV? I'm nineteen years old—I haven't even picked a major yet!" Evan's thoughts raced. He realized Dr. Litz had stopped talking and was waiting for him to open his eyes and look at her.

She slowed down her speech and made sure he was able to focus his attention back to the present. "Okay, I want you to really listen to what I'm saying. At this point, this only means that you have a positive test for HIV. It hopefully will prove to be a false positive, but we've got to send off more tests to figure that out. The awful part is that those confirmatory tests take over a week to get back, so you'll be in limbo wondering whether or not this is real. In the meantime, here's the bottom line. This HIV test that you took is designed to catch as many true positives as possible. Because of that, if you are in a low-risk population, the chance of a positive result being a false positive can be up to fifty percent. However, if you are in a high-risk group, then the likelihood of it being a true positive is actually very high. Our job right now is to go back over your history, and let's figure out if you are truly high or low risk, okay?"

Evan's brain was still spinning, but he nodded in agreement. He hadn't quite found his voice yet. Dr. Litz continued, "Now, Evan, I've got to ask you several questions that I should already know the answers to, but we need to be thorough. Have you ever used any IV drugs?"

"Yeah, right." He rolled his eyes. "No, never," he said, seeing in Dr. Litz's expression that this was no time for sarcasm.

"Have you ever had any sexual activity with another guy?" she asked.

This time, he gave a simple no.

"Okay, your first girlfriend that you had sex with—what was her name?"

"Courtney."

"That's right, Courtney. Now, as I recall, she was previously married and divorced, right?" she asked.

"Yes."

"Um, do you know if she had any other partners before her husband?"

"Yeah. She had one other high school boyfriend before James," Evan replied.

"Do we have any idea if that high school boyfriend had previous partners?"

"Not a clue."

"Okay, then, back to James, the ex-husband. What do we know about him?" Dr. Litz asked.

"That he's a jerk. And an addict," Evan snorted.

Dr. Litz's heart sank, but she tried to keep her voice steady. "What kind of addict? Did he use IV drugs?"

Evan shrugged. "I have no idea. Courtney referred to him as being an addict. I kind of assumed she meant pot, but now I'm not so sure. It never seemed important to ask."

"What about his sexual history?" asked the doctor.

Evan thought for a minute. "Well, I do know that he already has a new girlfriend, because unfortunately, they were apparently sleeping together while Courtney and I were supposed to be together. It turned out that Courtney was still occasionally sleeping with James, which is why we broke up," Josh replied.

"And the girlfriend? Do we have any clue?"

"No. But she's even older, like thirty, and I do know she has kids, so obviously she's had at least one other partner," Evan muttered.

Dr. Litz paused, then asked, "Did you have any discussions with Courtney about whether or not she'd had an STD or STD testing before?"

Evan thought for a minute, then replied, "You know, actually, she did get something from James once, but she commented that thank goodness one round of antibiotics cured whatever it was. In fact, that's how she found out originally that he was cheating on her when they were married."

"So, it sounds like James probably has had several partners?" the doctor asked quietly.

"Oh, man, I never thought about it that way before..." Evan sunk his head into his hands and rubbed his temples. "I'll bet he's had dozens of partners. Crap, why on earth didn't I think about this before? Dr. Litz, it's not fair, I'm *not* that way, and here I'm the one with... with a positive test." Evan couldn't bring himself to even say HIV yet.

Dr. Litz sadly shook her head and sighed. "You're absolutely right,

Evan, it isn't fair. You feel like you've only had sex with one person, but the truth is that you effectively sleep not just with that person, but with everyone that person has slept with, and so on and so on. Even if Courtney had only slept with two men, and each of them had slept with two other women, that would expose you to at least six other people just by sleeping with Courtney."

Evan interrupted, "And you can bet that James slept with a heck of a lot more than two women, and I highly doubt their virginity ...all of which means I'm screwed, doesn't it? Does this make me 'high risk'?"

Again, Dr. Litz shook her head. "Honestly, I'm not sure. We used to define high risk as anyone who had over six partners when it came to STDs. You can do the math that with six direct contacts, you're quickly into some very high numbers for exposure. The biggest problem here is that we're not sure about your secondary exposure. However, we do know that you don't have any of the other big risk factors—drug use or homosexual contact—so overall, I still think that there is a solid chance that this will turn out to be a false positive."

"So back to that false positive thing. Why would you use a test that can come back as a false positive half of the time? That doesn't make any sense to me," said Evan.

"No, no, that's not what I meant. A false positive actually occurs only once in about three hundred thousand tests. When there is a positive test result, if that person is truly low risk, that specific test has up to a fifty percent false positive rate. Does that make sense?"

"Um, no."

"Okay, let me give you another example. If you take a totally healthy, nonsmoking, thirty-something-year-old female runner and give her a stress treadmill test to look for heart disease, there is an extremely low chance of it being positive. However, if it is positive, it's more likely to be a false positive than a true positive because she has no risk factors for heart disease. Anyway, does that make more sense to you?" she asked.

"Yeah, actually, it does. So I either have HIV, or I'm the 'lucky winner' of a one in three hundred thousand chance of having a false positive. Great," Evan said sarcastically.

"Or, let's look at it that you can still have up to a fifty–fifty chance that it's not real. Let's leave the glass half full, okay?" smiled Dr. Litz.

"Easy for you to say. It's looking half empty from here. So what if it is real? Then what happens next?" he asked.

"Well, we get you right in with an infectious disease specialist, and they will decide whether or not you start on any antiviral drugs."

She thought for a minute, and then added, "Evan, do you know the difference between having HIV and having AIDS?"

"No, I really don't. Isn't it all the same?" he asked.

"Not at all. Many people are HIV positive but continue functioning perfectly well for years. It's not until the HIV has attacked and killed off most of the body's immune defenses that people develop the opportunistic infections that are diagnostic of AIDS. There are skin and respiratory infections that cannot take place in a healthy immune system and occur only when those defenses are shut down. When a person gets these specific infections, then they receive the diagnosis of AIDS."

"Okay, assuming I'm positive, Dr. Litz, how long am I going to live?" Evan took a deep breath and really focused on Dr. Litz.

"Evan, I don't have a crystal ball, but right now the time from diagnosis of HIV-positive antibodies until the onset of AIDS can be many years. We used to feel getting HIV was a death sentence, but now many people are leading productive lives and dealing with their HIV disease much like others deal with diabetes or any other chronic illness. I'm confident we'll continue to advance our research and improve our drugs, fighting both HIV itself and the infections that take over when the immune system is beat down. In fact, we can no longer even predict the average life expectancy from the diagnosis of AIDS because every year the numbers are improving."

Dr. Litz continued, "You might be wondering why in the heck I am telling you about this test before we know for sure one way or another. The biggest reason is that you told me this week that you are sleeping with a new girlfriend. Ethically, I absolutely had to tell you to minimize her risk. You don't get or give HIV from hugging, kissing, or sharing food, but you certainly can transmit it by sex. I'm glad you've been using condoms, but condoms can break, and if you are HIV positive, your new girlfriend needs to know. I know this is a ton to digest, but do you have any questions right now?" she asked.

"How long until we know for sure?"

"Roughly a week. Our lab sends your blood to California to run the Western blot test, which is a DNA test that takes several days to process. We'll also draw your blood again today to send off another test to check for the amount of virus in your blood, and that test should actually be back in a few days," she replied.

"So if the quicker test is negative?"

"That's great news, but we still wait for the Western blot DNA test to be one hundred percent sure," she replied.

Evan's brain was still racing; mainly he was furious with Courtney and wondering how quickly he could reach her by phone to grill her about her ex. Evan couldn't bear to think about Hanna. He could picture her beautiful innocent eyes filling with tears when he told her the news. Man, he would kill Courtney if this turned out to really be HIV. One in three hundred thousand...could he really be that unlucky? Of course, at this point, it would actually be lucky for it to turn out to be a false positive. If only there were a way to really know his risk.

Dr. Litz's voice interrupted his thoughts. "Evan?"

He looked up.

Dr. Litz smiled. "Evan, either way, we'll get through this." She handed him her business card. "Here are the best ways to reach me. I'm sure you'll have more questions later, so feel free to call back whenever. Is your cell phone the best way to reach you?"

"Absolutely. Please don't call my parents' home. They would totally freak out. I'm not going to tell them until we know for certain, okay?" he pleaded.

"Evan, don't worry. You're nineteen. Anything we discuss stays between us unless you ask me to tell them something. But you know, if you do want me to talk to your parents, I'd be happy to do so."

"Not now. Let's wait and see what the tests show this week. So, you'll call as soon as you hear?"

"I promise. The minute they fax me the results, I'll call you on your cell. I know how anxious you'll be. Let's try to stay optimistic, and I'll talk to you later this week. Okay?" she asked. Dr. Litz hoped her voice didn't reflect her true suspicions. The reality was that with Evan's secondary contacts, it sounded like he was not in the low-risk category, which meant that his Western blot test was likely to come back confirming HIV disease.

Evan took his lab slip and other paperwork from Dr. Litz. What a morning this had been. His hand gripped tightly the cell phone in his pocket. "Okay, Dr. Litz," he replied. He checked out and walked around the corner toward the lab. Before he went in to get his blood drawn, he stopped and leaned against the wall, feeling almost faint for a moment. As the magnitude of the whole thing began to really hit him, he pulled out his phone and hit "one" on his autodial. "Courtney" showed up on the screen as the call went through, and Evan practically erupted with rage when she answered his call with her casual, "Hey, Evan, glad you called. What's up?"

Gee, what's up? More than she ever expected.

15: Tanya

TANYA SMILED AT HER reflection in the mirror as she removed the extra earrings from her upper ears. Looking back at her was a polished, professional woman. Her long hair was slicked back in a tidy French knot, covering the tops of her ears and revealing only tasteful diamond stud earrings at the base of her earlobes. Tanya plucked a few cat hairs off the shoulder of her stylish navy blue suit. "I can't have animal hair messing up this perfect picture," she giggled.

Since she was old enough to remember, Tanya had taken in every stray or wounded animal that she found. From fallen baby birds to lost dogs or cats, Tanya loved to nurse them back to health and find new homes for them. Tanya's mom, an animal lover herself, supported Tanya's actions, but she set a rule that any animal brought in the house had a two-week grace period during which Tanya must find it a permanent home. As Tanya looked around her apartment at Sir Lance, her cat; Calypso, her parakeet; a tank full of fish; and her old dog, Shadow, she could see the wisdom in that rule.

Tanya thought wistfully of her mom. "If only you could see me now, Mom," she mused, "I look so conservative, you'd think I vote Republican." Her mom had died, still worrying about Tanya's future, before Tanya had finished college. If she could only see her former "wild child" starting a job as a full-fledged certified public accountant, she would be at peace.

Tanya had rebelled during her first couple of years in college. "Your friends look like the strays that we've always taken in," her mother had commented more than once.

Tanya would immediately defend her companions. "Mom, their clothes are vintage, and you should be impressed that they shop at thrift shops rather than spending a ton of money on high-end fashion."

Her father's words were significantly harsher. "Tanya, you'll be judged by the company you keep. Young people dressed head-to-toe in black and smoking cigarettes don't impress anyone, and you befriending these drug addicts isn't noble—it's stupid. Don't call me to bail you out of jail."

"They're not drug addicts," Tanya had protested, but in truth, the crowd she hung out with not only partied hard with alcohol and cigarettes, but most of them routinely experimented with other drugs "to help get their creative juices flowing."

Over half of the group was involved in theater, and they carried their flair for the dramatic off the stage and into their everyday life. Constant political and social debates challenged many of Tanya's childhood beliefs. Late-night arguments about the need to legalize marijuana offered Tanya new perspectives on what had previously been a black-and-white issue to her. Perhaps the most startling behavior to Tanya was their acceptance of casual sex partners within the group, which they referred to as "friends with benefits."

Tanya began to experiment with her appearance, adding several ear piercings and a belly-button ring, reveling in the freedom of this self-expression. Eventually she even got a small tattoo of a dove but placed it in an easily concealed location over her right shoulder blade. Her family worried about her external changes, fearing that she was headed down a path of self-destruction. However, while

Tanya's ideas had liberalized a bit, her actions remained very conservative within this social group, as she never indulged beyond a couple of beers or a glass of wine.

Tanya's thoughts turned briefly to Devon, her first serious boyfriend and the dominant personality in the group. Devon had grown up traveling around the world with his father's oil business. Tall and slender, with thick jet-black hair and a vaguely British accent, Devon had enchanted Tanya from the moment they met. She was fascinated with his sophisticated ideals and zest for life. Tanya dated him exclusively for nearly two years, despite the fact that he openly continued to see other women. Tanya had naively thought that if she could make him love her enough, he wouldn't need others to satisfy his desires. After giving up her virginity, emotional innocence, and two years of her life, Tanya moved on to more mutually beneficial relationships during the rest of college.

At this point, Tanya was decidedly happy to be single. It had taken all of her time and energy throughout the last year to study for and pass the CPA exam, and she was excited for today, her first real day of work. The last few weeks had been considered orientation to the firm, covering all different areas of accounting as well as explanations of their benefits, from retirement plans to health and life insurance policies. Today Tanya would finally start in the audit section, her main area of interest. She gave Shadow a pat on his head, freshened up the water bowls, fed the fish, and headed out the door.

Tanya looked around as she slid through the revolving door at the entrance of her building. "No matter how you slice it, I'm definitely grown up now," she thought, as she headed towards the elevator bank.

"Hey, Tanya," said a deep voice behind her.

"Good morning, Jim," Tanya replied with pleasure. Jim had made it a point to sit next to her during orientation the week before. His new suit complemented his tall, athletic frame. "Nice threads," Tanya added coyly.

"You clean up pretty well yourself," Jim smiled. "Are you nervous about getting started today?"

"Does it show?" Tanya laughed.

"Actually, no, that's why I asked," replied Jim. "I was hoping I wasn't the only one worked up over finally getting started."

"Well, I'm ready, nervous or not. At least now I'll be doing what interests me, instead of all that tax stuff we had to suffer through last week," said Tanya.

"So how about if you and I grab dinner and drinks tonight to celebrate the end of our first real day?" Jim smoothly requested.

Tanya paused for a moment, shouting inside her head, "Sweet!" but out loud saying, "You know, that would be great. Where should we meet?"

"How about here in the lobby at five ten?" suggested Jim, as they entered the elevator together.

"Five ten it is," agreed Tanya, noting to herself that only two accountants would pick such a specific time.

The day sped by quickly, and Tanya was deeply engrossed in her work late in the morning when her supervisor approached her with a message. "Tanya, they want to see you downstairs in the main office. They said it's something about your orientation paperwork and to head down now to take care of it."

"Okay," consented Tanya, wondering what could be missing from her file, as she had been compulsive about completing the mountain of forms that they had been given. Tanya walked into the reception area and gave her name to the secretary. "Oh yes, I have your notice right here," said the cheerful woman, handing her a sealed envelope. Tanya took it and headed back toward her floor, opening the letter and scanning it quickly as she waited for the elevator. Tanya's eyes skipped down the form letter until she saw the reason for the notice. "Please call Dr. Andrews to follow up on abnormal lab results from your life insurance screening physical."

"Well, that's odd," mused Tanya, "I feel perfectly fine." She went back to her desk and decided she'd make the phone call before she delved back into her work.

"Health Partners, how may I help you?" answered a receptionist.

"Hi, this is Tanya Leslie, and I'm a new employee at Abbott Accounting. I received a note that I apparently had some abnormal bloodwork on my screening tests and that I should call for an appointment."

"Oh, well, you're in luck, because I just had a cancellation for an afternoon appointment today at three. Can you make that? We're right down the street from your firm. Otherwise, he's booked for about a week."

Tanya realized that today was likely better than next week, when she would be fully involved in her work, so she consented. "That would be fine."

"Great. Please come fifteen minutes early to fill out paperwork, and bring your insurance card."

Tanya hung up the phone, cleared the afternoon appointment with her supervisor, and resumed her work. "Oh great, this looks brilliant," Tanya thought sarcastically, "a few hours into my first day at work, and I'm asking off. I'm in perfect health, and now it looks like I'm some slacker."

At exactly two forty-five, Tanya sat in the doctor's office, completing her new patient forms. "When you answer 'no' to all the questions, it doesn't take fifteen minutes to fill these out," she mused. The forms asked about past surgeries, hospitalizations, pregnancies, and past diseases from asthma to sexually transmittable diseases. "The only 'yes' I have is a recent tetanus shot, from when a neighborhood cat had accidentally scratched me," reflected Tanya. She turned in her forms and was promptly transferred back to an exam room. Tanya glanced at her watch, pleased that perhaps she would be back to work quickly. Unfortunately, it was almost three thirty when the doctor finally walked into her exam room, wearing a somber expression on his face.

"Tanya Leslie? I'm Dr. Andrews," said the short, balding physician dressed in a dated coat and tie.

"Hello, nice to meet you," replied Tanya, returning his firm handshake.

"I see from your paperwork that you've been relatively healthy," he began.

"The only time I've been sick in the past five years is when I had mononucleosis my sophomore year in college," agreed Tanya.

"Did they do a blood test?" asked the doctor.

"I honestly don't remember," said Tanya. "I had a fever and a sore throat. They said it was not strep throat and that it was likely mono.

There were a ton of students on campus with mono that semester."

"And since then, you've been pretty healthy?" followed up Dr. Andrews.

"Since I quit hanging around with smokers, I haven't even had a cold," assured Tanya. "Why are you asking all this? What did my test show that could have you look so concerned?"

Dr. Andrews's smile faded, and he took a deep breath. "Tanya, there's no good way to tell you this. Your HIV test came back positive, and it's been confirmed with two additional tests. The first test is a called an EIA test, and it is automatically repeated if there is a positive. After two positives, we send off for a second, more definitive, test called a Western blot. All of your tests were positive."

Tanya's mouth dropped open in disbelief. "HIV? Are you telling me I have AIDS? That's impossible."

"No, you do not have AIDS, but you do have HIV disease. The rest of your lab tests look great, though. You're not anemic, and your white blood cell count is strong."

"Wait a second," interrupted Tanya, "what is the difference between HIV disease and AIDS? Aren't they the same? This doesn't make any sense to me. And I don't feel bad."

"HIV disease means you are infected with the human immunodeficiency virus. AIDS, which stands for acquired immune deficiency syndrome, refers to the very advanced stage of HIV disease, when the immune system is so damaged that it can't fight off many infections," explained the doctor. "It's great that you appear so healthy otherwise. With all the new medicines that we have to fight HIV, I hope you'll stay that way for a long time."

"I'm sorry," Tanya protested, raising both hands, palms out, in front of her. "There has to be a mistake. I've never done IV drugs, and I'm not promiscuous. I've only had sex with a few guys in my entire life, and none of them were gay or bisexual. I'm not sick. Isn't it far more likely that your test is wrong? I simply don't believe this. Please, why don't we draw my blood again today, and if it comes back positive again, then I'll deal with this, okay? I'll bet my blood sample got switched with someone else's in the lab or something."

"Look, I have to tell you that I do believe these test results are accurate, but I'm happy to follow your suggestion and repeat the test today. I know that this is a lot to absorb, and I've got no doubt that you are a clean-cut young lady. Unfortunately, having sex with anyone, even one guy, is a risk, because you don't know for certain his entire past sexual history. HIV disease is not restricted to homosexuals, prostitutes, or IV drug users," lectured Dr. Andrews. "What did you use for protection?"

"I was on the pill," replied Tanya.

"So you didn't think you needed to use condoms?" he asked.

Tanya bit her lip, shaking her head in the negative, and firmly refusing to believe that she could have contracted HIV. "No, it's impossible," she decided, "but if I did, it would have to be Devon, Mr. 'I-can't-limit-myself-to-one-person.' When was the last time anyone heard about him? Matt had definitely been a virgin, and Jeff had only a couple of old girlfriends, so it had to be Devon..." Tanya's thoughts raced on, but she realized the doctor had been talking and seemed to be waiting for an answer. "I'm sorry, could you repeat that?" Tanya mumbled apologetically.

"I was saying that if this test confirms the others, we'll get you an appointment with Dr. Knorr, the infectious disease specialist. There are so many new drug protocols that I generally leave it up to the specialist to establish your drug regimen. Do you have any other questions for me right now?" asked Dr. Andrews.

"HIV can't be spread by kissing someone, right?" inquired Tanya.

"Correct. HIV is only spread through direct contact of blood or body fluids from an infected person, such as through oral, vaginal, or anal sex, or by sharing needles. Casual contact like hugging and kissing does not transmit the virus," he responded.

Dr. Andrews examined Tanya, looking in her mouth, eyes, and ears, feeling her neck, and listening to her heart and lungs. "Everything looks good," he reassured Tanya. "Let's recheck your bloodwork, and we should have the results in a couple days. How would you like us to contact you with the results?"

"Please call my cell phone. I wrote it on my paperwork as my primary contact number," Tanya replied somewhat curtly.

Shortly after the doctor exited the room, a short, middle-aged brunette walked in. "Tanya? I'm Cindy, the phlebotomist for Health Partners. Looks like we need to repeat a blood test for you."

Tanya felt her face turning beet red. "I have to tell you, I'm sure that last test was a mistake. I'm perfectly healthy," she assured Cindy. Nonetheless, it seemed to Tanya that Cindy took more care drawing her blood than the previous lab technician had.

"This might sting a bit, please don't move or pull away," Cindy said when she was ready to insert the needle. Once the blood was drawn, Cindy very quickly and cautiously disposed of the needle and then sealed the tube of blood inside a Ziploc-style bag and placed a bandage on Tanya before removing and disposing of her gloves in a red canister marked "biohazard."

"Could I feel any more like a leper?" thought Tanya, inwardly cringing away from Cindy's defensive body language. "What if I really do have HIV? Is this how people are going to act around me? Will everyone be afraid of me?"

"Okay, you can check out down the hall with the receptionist," Cindy was saying, dismissing Tanya.

Tanya left the doctor's office, and automatically began walking back down the street to her office. She glanced at her watch. "It's four ten. Okay, I have to hold it together for less than an hour before I can head home and figure this out," Tanya thought. And then, her heart sinking, she remembered Jim. "Was that only this morning that I was so excited to accept his dinner invitation? There is absolutely no way that I can go out with him tonight and act normal. I'm going to blow this relationship before it even gets started," she whined to herself. "Of course, if I've got HIV, that's not exactly going to help any relationship to take off," her practical side added.

Back at work, she robotically resumed her tasks, pushing all other thoughts out of her head. At precisely ten after five, Tanya met Jim in the lobby and excused herself from dinner, blaming a family crisis that had popped up in the afternoon and agreeing to reschedule dinner for next week.

She maintained composure until she collapsed onto her couch at home, Shadow thrusting his paws onto her lap and Sir Lance pacing back and forth along the top of the couch behind her head. First silent tears, then heaving sobs racked Tanya as she tried to process the possibility of having HIV disease. "What will my family say? Dad will want to strangle Devon, if not me. What will my friends think?

Should I tell anyone at work? Oh my God, what if I gave it to Matt or Jeff? How will I live with myself? Why didn't I use condoms? Would it have mattered? Should I try to reach Devon? How could I have been so stupid?"

Rapid-fire questions cycled endlessly in her brain, with no answers to be found. Eventually she would decide the whole thing was ridiculous, and that this angst was for nothing. Then the questions would start again, sending her into a downward spiral. By the time the phone call came two days later, Tanya felt emotionally drained.

"This is Tanya," she said, her heart pounding as she answered the call from Health Partners.

"Tanya, this is Lori, Dr. Andrews's nurse," said a kind voice. "I'm sorry, but the repeat HIV test is still positive. Dr. Andrews asked me to help you set up an appointment with the infectious disease specialist. I called them, and they can work you in tomorrow morning at ten thirty. Can you make that time?"

Tanya could barely speak. "Um, yes, thank you." She wrote down the office address and phone number, completely in shock.

"Feel free to call us if you have any problems," Lori was saying.

"Sure," Tanya hissed.

"Tanya, I'm so sorry. It'll be okay, though. Dr. Knorr is the best. She'll take good care of you," Lori said empathetically.

"I'm sorry, too," concurred Tanya, ending the call. "Believe me, I'm deeply sorry."

facts

HIV Fact Sheet

What is it?

- HIV stands for human immunodeficiency virus, the virus that causes AIDS (acquired immune deficiency syndrome).

How common is it?

- More than 1 million Americans have confirmed HIV infection or AIDS.

- The CDC believes that up to 25% of infected people in the United States do not know they are infected.

- An estimated 40,000 Americans are newly infected each year.

- According to the CDC, AIDS is seven times more prevalent in African Americans and three times more prevalent in Hispanic Americans than in Caucasian Americans.

- 2006 data shows 35,314 newly diagnosed cases of HIV/AIDS, 74% male and 26% female.

How do you get it?

- HIV is transmitted by direct contact between an infected person's blood or body fluids with another person's blood, broken skin, or mucous membranes; therefore, HIV is transmitted by sex (oral, anal, or vaginal) or sharing needles or syringes (which may occur with IV drug use).

- 2006 data shows that 80% of women and 16% of men with newly diagnosed HIV/AIDS contracted the disease through high-risk heterosexual contact (meaning having sex with someone who has HIV or is at high risk—an IV drug user or a man who has sex with men).

- Pregnant mothers infected with HIV can transmit the virus to their unborn child during pregnancy, delivery, or breastfeeding.

Where on your body do you get it?

- HIV infects white blood cells, specifically the CD4+T cells. HIV infection itself is not visible on the outside of the body.

How do I know if I have it?

- Many people are asymptomatic, on average for up to ten years after the initial infection.

- Some people get a flu-like illness within the first few months of infection. They develop headache, fever, fatigue, and enlarged lymph nodes.

- Blood tests can detect antibodies to HIV, whether or not people have any symptoms. There are three tests: the EIA (enzyme immunoassay)—a rapid screening test—or the Western blot or an IFA (immunofluorescence assay), slower, confirmatory tests.

- Late in the disease, when the immune system is weakened, other symptoms begin to appear, such as frequent yeast infections, unusual rashes, fevers and sweats, weight loss, severe herpes infections, and/or short-term memory loss.

What does it look like?

- While there are some characteristic skin lesions late in the disease, most people with HIV infection look completely normal.

What does it feel like?

- Initially, many people feel tired or have unexplained weight loss, fevers, or chills.

- Lymph nodes may swell and ache (in neck, armpits, or groin).

- Headache, muscle aches, stiff neck, sore throat, fever, and flu-like symptoms may occur within the first few months.

- Many people feel normal and are unaware that they are infected.

How long does it last?

- HIV infections currently last for a lifetime.

Can it be cured?

- Not yet, although treatments are improving every year.

Can HIV be transmitted between homosexual partners?

- 50% of HIV-infected individuals in the United States are men who have sex with men (per 2006 CDC data).

- There are case reports of woman-to-woman transmission, likely involving menstrual blood or vaginitis, but the rate of transmission is unknown.

What is AIDS?

- AIDS, or acquired immune deficiency syndrome, refers to the most advanced stage of HIV infection. There are set criteria to define it, including blood counts (CD4+T cells < 200), and the presence of at least 1 of 26 infections that wouldn't typically be present in a person with a healthy immune system.

- 2006 data shows that for untreated HIV disease, the time from initial HIV infection until the development of AIDS can range from a few months to 17 years, with the median time being 10 years.

What is the treatment?

- Antiviral medicines called reverse transcriptase inhibitors block the virus from copying itself.

- There are over three main classes of drugs, but because HIV can easily become resistant to medicines, HIV disease is usually treated with a combination of drugs, which is more effective.

- Other medicines are added to prevent opportunistic infections (bacterial, viral, and parasitic infections that generally don't make people with normal immune systems ill).

- There can be serious side effects from any of the anti-HIV drugs, so patients must work closely with their doctors to ensure optimal care.

Is there a vaccine?

- Vaccines are undergoing clinical trials but are not available for general use yet.

How about alternative therapies?

- No alternative medicine therapies can cure HIV infection. Vitamin and mineral supplementation is the most prevalent alternative medicine practice among HIV+ individuals.

- Exercise, including resistance training to build muscle, is encouraged.

- Meditation, yoga, massage, and herbal medicines are also being used to complement conventional treatments.

Are there long-term consequences?

- HIV progresses to AIDS, which results in fatality from opportunistic infections and cancers.

When are you contagious?

- Always.

How do I avoid getting HIV?

- Abstinence from IV drug use or sharing needles and from vaginal, anal, and oral sex will prevent the transmission of HIV.

- Proper use of condoms decreases transmission of HIV.

- Use fresh condoms with each partner if sharing sex toys, or preferably, do not share sex toys.

- If you are in the healthcare profession, take extra care to avoid contaminated needle sticks (including but not limited to wearing gloves and not recapping needles).

- Limit sexual intimacy to a monogamous relationship in which both parties have tested negative for HIV at least six months after their last sexual contact (or after their other high-risk behavior, such as sharing needles).

If I have HIV, how do I avoid giving it to my partner?

- The only way to be 100% sure not to transmit HIV is to abstain from oral, vaginal, and anal sex and from sharing needles.

Frequently Asked Questions

➤ **Can you catch HIV from hugging, kissing, or shaking hands with someone who is infected?**
No. The virus dies when it dries out.

➤ **Can you catch HIV from a toilet seat?**
No. HIV dies quickly once it is outside the body.

➤ **Can you catch HIV from sharing a drinking glass or water fountain?**
No. The virus can be detected in saliva, but there is no evidence that it can be transmitted by saliva.

➤ **Can you catch HIV today from a blood transfusion?**
No. Since 1985, all donated blood in the United States has been tested for HIV antibodies. If you received a blood transfusion prior to 1985, however, you could be at risk.

➤ **Don't you have to be gay or abuse drugs to catch HIV?**
No. The 2006 data from the CDC shows that while 67% of men newly infected with HIV had male-to-male sexual contact, 12% reported IV drug use, and 5% had male-to-male sexual contact and injection drug use, 16% had only heterosexual contact and did not use IV drugs.

The same data source shows that 80% of women newly infected reported only heterosexual contact and no IV drug use (with another 19% reporting IV drug use).

An increasing number of men are reported to be on the "down low," meaning they profess to be purely heterosexual but engage in male-to-male sexual activities in addition to heterosexual ones.

Additional Information

AIDSinfo
P. O. Box 6303
Rockville, MD 20849-6303
1-800-HIV-0440 (1-800-448-0440), or 301-519-0459
1-888-480-3739 TTY/TDD
http://aidsinfo.nih.gov

American College of Obstetricians and Gynecologists
P. O. Box 96920
409 12th Street, SW
Washington, DC 20090-6920
202-863-2518
www.acog.org/publications/patient_education/bp082.cfm

American Social Health Association
P. O. Box 13827
Research Triangle Park, NC 27709
1-800-227-8922
www.ashastd.org/learn/learn_hiv_aids.cfm

CDC-INFO
Centers for Disease Control and Prevention
1600 Clifton Road
Atlanta, GA 30333
1-800-CDC-INFO (1-800-232-4636), 1-888-232-6348 TTY
www.cdc.gov/hiv/

MedlinePlus
National Library of Medicine
8600 Rockville Pike
Bethesda, MD 20894
1-888-FIND-NLM (1-888-346-3656), or 301-594-5983
www.nlm.nih.gov/medlineplus/aids.html

HEPATITIS C

16: Jane

JANE RUSHED INTO the house with her arms full, stumbling over the daily batch of mail. She unloaded the groceries, grabbed a snack for the kids, gathered up the mail, and jumped back into her car, heading over to school to pick up her kids and deliver them to their respective activities. When the last child, Cory, left the car for his trumpet lesson, she glanced at the mail and noticed an official-looking letter from the blood bank. As Jane slid open the envelope, she privately congratulated herself, thinking that this would likely be a thank-you note for her contribution to the church's annual blood drive.

Jane had been excited to give blood for the first time in her life this year. The blood bank had just decreased their minimum weight requirement for donors from 110 lbs. to 105, so Jane was finally eligible to give the "gift of life." At five foot one (okay, five feet and half an inch, but who's counting?) the former cheerleader turned thirty-eight-year-old PTA president still looked as though she might be a recent college graduate. Strawberry blond hair, freckles, and dimples completed her cherubic appearance, thanks to her Irish roots. Jane had such positive energy and enthusiasm that she never lacked for volunteers for any project, no matter how onerous the task. She was the first one to jump in and roll up her sleeves to get a job done, and it had always bothered her that she was ineligible to donate blood when she organized the semi-annual blood drive. Jane smiled as she opened her letter and began to read:

> Dear Mrs. Jane Mahoney,
> Thank you for your recent donation to the Travis County Blood Bank. Unfortunately, we are unable to use your blood, as it tested positive for hepatitis C. Please see your primary care physician for further evaluation.

Jane's first thought was sheer disappointment. "I finally gave blood, and they couldn't even use it? What a bummer," she mused. As she sat there feeling sorry for herself, her mind began processing the rest of the information. "Now wait a minute," she thought. "Hepatitis C? What on earth is that—some kind of food poisoning? I did have oysters a few weeks ago. Isn't that what causes hepatitis?"

Jane was puzzled, especially since she hadn't been sick at all. Oh well, she thought, maybe it's a mistake. I guess it's time to call our family doctor, Dr. Wren, and go in to have an annual exam. Jane realized, as she thought about it, that since she had had her tubes tied after the extremely difficult pregnancy with the twins, she had slacked off on getting her yearly physicals. When she was having babies, her gynecologist did her exams. However, since Marlee and Millette were born, Jane had only made time for one or two physicals in the last six years. She grabbed her cell phone, called information, and was soon connected with the receptionist at the doctor's office.

"Hi. This is Jane Mahoney, and I'd like to make an appointment with Dr. Wren."

"Okay. Did you have any special concerns, or is this just your routine visit?" inquired the receptionist.

"Well, I am definitely overdue for my annual exam, and I just received a letter from the blood bank saying I've got some kind of hepatitis, so that's why I'm calling now," Jane replied casually.

"Hepatitis? Oh, that really shouldn't wait until your physical. Dr. Wren is booked up for a couple months for routine annuals. Let's go ahead and make you an appointment soon for the hepatitis, and then we'll plug you in for your physical in February, okay?"

"Well, I'm not sick or anything. Can't everything just wait until February?" Jane nervously inquired, and apprehension spawned butterflies in her stomach.

"Actually, no. I'm glad you're feeling well, but I think Dr. Wren would want to see you sooner to discuss your hepatitis. In fact, we have an acute care spot open tomorrow morning at ten. Will that work for you?"

Jane grabbed her day planner and looked at Friday's schedule. "Um, ten will be fine. Is this something I need to be concerned about?" she asked.

"Don't worry, Dr. Wren will be able to answer all your questions at your appointment tomorrow. Please be here fifteen minutes early to fill out paperwork, and remember to bring your current insurance card. It looks like you've not been in for a while. Are you still on Blue Cross insurance?"

Jane fumbled through her purse for her insurance card and gave the receptionist all her vital statistics. She was still giving out information when Cory startled her by jumping in the car and slamming the car door as he tossed his trumpet onto the car seat.

"Hey, what's for dinner? I'm starved," he announced.

Jane finished up her phone call and jotted down the appointment time in her planner. "How was your lesson?" she asked as they pulled away.

The rest of the evening passed in a blur as she gathered the kids from their activities and managed to get everyone fed, showered, and ready for bed just as her husband, Will, arrived home late from a business meeting.

As they shared a glass of wine together during their nightly ritual of chatting about their day, Jane mentioned the letter and her doctor's appointment to Will. "So, do you think I got this hepatitis from those oysters we ate last month?" Jane asked.

"Honestly, honey, I have no idea. I thought hepatitis C was something that drug addicts got," Will said, without thinking.

"Well, is this the first time you've given blood?"

"Yes."

"And did Will give blood this year, too?"

"Yes, and he didn't get any letter, if that's where you're headed," replied Jane.

"And, basically, you've been healthy? No nausea, diarrhea, or un-explained fatigue?" she asked.

"I'm afraid all my fatigue is perfectly explainable," Jane smiled.

"Well, let's take a look at you, then," Dr. Wren said as she reached for her stethoscope. She looked Jane over head to toe, only paus-ing for a moment during her exam of Jane's abdomen. She pointed to Jane's lower right belly. "Remind me. What's the story behind this?"

Jane flushed, instinctively reaching up to cover her tattoo. "You know, what am I going to say to my kids when they want a tattoo? Now I know why my mom freaked out when I got this shamrock. She kept telling me that I would regret it when I was older. I have to tell you, though; it seemed awfully cool when I got it. Our senior year, all the cheerleaders wanted to have some permanent reminder of our year. Everyone thought we were such 'goody-goodies,' and we kind of wanted to do something rebellious. On our senior spring break trip, we decided to go together and each get a tasteful, small tattoo that would just barely show above our biki-nis. Almost all of us went through with it, and I picked a shamrock because I was headed to Notre Dame. At least we decided on a spot that wouldn't be visible with regular clothes on. Who thought back then how it would look after it got stretched out a few times with having kids?"

Dr. Wren smiled. "Well, it's still cute, even if one side got a bit stretched out. My only concern about it is that, apparently, it's your only risk factor for hepatitis C."

Jane was shocked. "You mean, you can catch it from getting a tat-too? This tattoo is over twenty years old. Wouldn't it have showed up before now?"

Dr. Wren shook her head. "Not necessarily. Do you remember anything about the shop where you got it? I doubt back then that you asked if they sterilized their needles."

"Oh my gosh, no, I have no idea. We thought it looked like a decent place, but it never occurred to any of us that getting a tattoo could be a health risk. Do you really think that's how I got this?"

"Well, assuming that our repeat test today confirms that you really do have hepatitis C, that would be my educated guess. There is some debate in the medical literature about how often it is transmitted that way, but it is a blood-borne disease, so it makes sense to me. Even if they used fresh needles, if they used the same ink for multiple people, it would be contaminated. Having said that, there are many people with hepatitis C that have no obvious risk factors, including tattoos."

"What about my husband, Will? Wouldn't he have it by now if I have had this for over twenty years?" asked Jane. "And oh my gosh, what about the kids? Could I have given it to them? They've never had any occasion to have their blood drawn." Jane was starting to panic. Her family was absolutely the most important thing in the world to her, and the thought that she could have harmed them was almost too much for her to tolerate.

Dr. Wren put her hand on Jane's arm. "Okay, one step at a time. Why don't I let you get dressed, and I'll be right back with some handouts about hepatitis C. It's possible that this was a false positive, but even if you do have it, chances are good that no one else in your family is infected. I promise we'll go over everything, okay?"

By the time Jane was dressed and feeling more composed, Dr. Wren was back. "Okay, Jane. The first thing we need to do is to draw your blood today and do another test to confirm whether or not you are truly infected. In the blood-donor population, a positive test can turn out to be wrong up to twenty percent of the time."

"Really?" Jane asked hopefully.

"Yes, however, let me go ahead and tell you about hepatitis, in case you are truly infected." She handed Jane an information sheet. "Let's go over this together, okay? First of all, there are different kinds of hepatitis. Hepatitis means inflammation of the liver. It can be infectious, like from hepatitis A, B, or C, or even from another virus such as mono. It can also come from alcoholism or medicines. We worry about hepatitis the most when it becomes chronic, meaning that the inflammation in the liver doesn't go away after the initial illness. With hepatitis C, many people don't remember being ill. The symptoms of early infection can be mild or are often like a case of food poisoning or a stomach virus, with several days of nausea, vomiting, or diarrhea. Then it can be silent for years, not noticed until there is enough inflammation to cause a rise in blood levels of liver enzymes."

"Like I had with my gallstones?" Jane interrupted.

"Yes. It is those same enzymes. We'll be checking those today, along with the repeat test for hepatitis C, to get an idea of how much inflammation you have. We'll also check to see if you have antibodies to hepatitis A and B, and we'll give you immunizations for those if you don't, to avoid any preventable further insult to your liver. Your kids are already immunized for hepatitis A and B, by the way. Routine vaccination of kids for hepatitis B began in 1991, and your kids received the hepatitis A vaccine when there was an outbreak in their daycare center. We don't have a shot yet to prevent hepatitis C. If you have had hepatitis C for all these years, your kids have a less than five percent chance of having caught it from you when you were pregnant. I know you breastfed them, too, and I want to reassure you that hepatitis C is not thought to be transmitted through breast milk."

"Thank goodness for that," said Jane.

Dr. Wren continued, "What we worry about with hepatitis C is that a percentage of people—somewhere between five and twenty percent—go on to develop scarring of the liver, called cirrhosis, and some even go on to develop liver cancer. Hepatitis C is the leading cause for liver transplantation. We do have treatments to prevent the progression of disease, but there are significant side effects to those treatments. Hopefully, you'll have only the hepatitis antibodies, with minimal liver inflammation, and we will just be able check your liver functions regularly without putting you on any medicines."

"So, what else do I need to do? Is there any special diet I need to follow?" asked Jane.

"Generally, we just want you to maximize your health. Eat right, exercise, and limit alcohol as much as possible. Also, we'll have you avoid acetaminophen, which is the brand name Tylenol, as a pain reliever, since it can irritate the liver," replied Dr. Wren.

"So goodbye to wine with dinner."

"At least as a regular event, yes," said Dr. Wren.

"But I'm not contagious if I'm kissing the kids or anything?" Jane asked.

"Really, it's just spread by blood. You shouldn't share razors or toothbrushes with anyone, but otherwise, it's not that contagious. You don't spread it by general close contact."

"Okay. What about Will? Should we be using condoms? That would certainly be ironic after being married this long and having my tubes tied," Jane said.

"In this setting, I wouldn't necessarily recommend that. As you've said, he's potentially been exposed for over two decades. Studies show that in long-term monogamous couples in which only one person is positive for hepatitis C, the transmission rate is less than one percent per year."

"And do we test him and the kids?"

Dr. Wren smiled. "If your test confirms this, then yes, we will test them all, but remember, the chances of the children being infected as well is very low. We should have your results early next week, and we'll call you as soon as we have them. Any other questions?"

"I guess not. I hope this shamrock has some Irish luck left in it," Jane said.

The phone call came Tuesday morning. Dr. Wren's nurse was pleasant enough, but the information was not. The second tests confirmed hepatitis C, but at least her liver enzyme levels were only mildly elevated. The doctor wanted her to make a follow-up appointment to discuss the results. Jane hung up the phone, somewhat in shock. "All of this, from a tattoo?" she thought. "Maybe moms *are* always right."

17: Luke

LUKE PUSHED BACK FROM his desk, swiveling in his soft leather chair to better absorb the spectacular view from his home office's picture window. Mount Crested Butte's sheer cliffs were beginning to cast shadows from the setting sun. Looking closely, Luke could make out the proud profile of an Indian chief's face along the far southern edge, where the rocky landslides met the aspens. The cool weather and shorter days were coaxing the aspens to become golden yellow, glistening between the evergreens.

"I can't believe I'm finally free to spend a whole month in the fall up here," Luke gloated. Luke was the president of his own startup software company. As long as he had good Internet access, he was free to travel away from his native San Jose, California. Throughout his twenties and early thirties, Luke had hopped flights to Crested Butte any time he could put together a three-day weekend. In the summer, he learned to whitewater raft and kayak. In the spring, Luke hit the single-track in this birthplace of mountain biking. For the two weeks of the fall color change, though, it was all about hiking. From Green Lake Trail to West Maroon Pass, Luke explored every open trail, inhaling the crisp scents and perfecting digital photographs of the aspens as they evolved.

When his company had gone public, Luke made millions of dollars. That happened four years ago, and his only major splurge was this new home in Crested Butte. Located on the back nine of the golf course, it gave him a view of town from one side of his house and this amazing view of the mountain from the other. The home was finished with high-end amenities, from a drop-down big-screen television to a climate-controlled walk-in wine cellar. "Life simply doesn't get any better than this," Luke said to his faithful companion, Stash, a three-year-old Labrador mix, who wagged his tail enthusiastically in agreement.

"Ellen would be awfully jealous of our wine collection, although she wouldn't fully appreciate the rest of the town," mused Luke. Ellen was Luke's last girlfriend. They had a brief but intense six-month relationship that had been a fun diversion, but Luke didn't miss her. Ellen was actually his former accountant. Shortly after Luke's company went public, Ellen had blindsided Luke by showing up unannounced at his condo with a bottle of wine to celebrate his newfound success. Unfortunately, it turned out that their only common interest was the profits from his company. Ellen enjoyed museums, fine dining, and shopping. Luke favored outdoor recreation, pizza, and beer. Luke gained an appreciation for excellent wine during the brief relationship but realized he preferred the easygoing companionship of a dog over complex human interaction.

Luke refocused on the task at hand. "Let me get through this last forwarded stack of mail, and we'll head out for a hike, okay, Stash?" he said to the dog. He turned back to the desk and picked up his aspen-handled letter opener, slitting open the remaining few envelopes as Stash bounded over by his side. "Stanford wants money again," he said, tossing his alma mater's request aside. "Another credit card offer we don't need," Luke commented about the second one, tossing it in the trash. "Looks like this is my new life insurance approval, Stash. Maybe I'll make you my beneficiary," Luke chuckled at the dog.

"Wait, what's this? Apparently, they don't like my liver, Stash. I need to have further tests and clearance from my regular doctor. I bet I can get in to see Dr. Joanne this week. Of course, we know what she's going to say, don't we, buddy?" said Luke, scratching his dog behind the ears. Stash licked Luke's hand and barked. "That's right, Stash. She's going to tell me to stop drinking. Oh well, I'll call for an appointment tomorrow."

Luke had seen a local doctor, Dr. Joanne, for a variety of minor ailments over the years. She had treated a broken arm from snowboarding, road rashes from mountain-bike crashes, and a few episodes of alcohol-related gastritis. He walked out of the study without another thought regarding his health and grabbed the leash. "Come on, let's go hike the upper loop."

A couple of days later, Luke had his appointment with Dr. Joanne to get her opinion on the abnormal liver tests. After examining him, the doctor sat across from Luke, flipping through the back of his chart and comparing the new numbers to the last lab results in his chart.

"Luke, looking back over the sporadic labs we have on you for the last seven or eight years, I only see one other time when your liver functions were abnormal. Three years ago, when you came in with stomach pain, your enzymes were elevated, but it looks like the tests were never repeated as I had suggested. Knowing you, you went back to California and forgot about it," she chastised.

"Well, I'm here for a whole month this time, so you should be able to fix me up, right Dr. Joanne?" he countered.

"We'll see. Let's go over a few things. Are you having nausea, vomiting, diarrhea, or pain?" she asked.

"Not at all," Luke reassured her.

"How about your reflux? Are you having any heartburn?" asked the doctor.

"You know, it comes and goes, but it hasn't been bad recently," admitted Luke. "I've been taking some antacids but no prescription medicines, like before."

"And you're not taking any medicines on a regular basis, including over-the-counter stuff like Tylenol, right?" she asked.

"No, I don't like pills, so I rarely even take an aspirin," Luke answered.

"How much alcohol are you drinking these days?" the doctor inquired.

"More than you'd approve of," said Luke, with a grin.

"Seriously, how many drinks per week?"

"During the week, most days I'll have a beer or a couple glasses of wine with dinner, but I'll admit that on the weekends, I may have more in a night if I'm out listening to music."

"And how's your caffeine? Still measuring by the pots?" asked Dr. Joanne.

"I switched to decaf for awhile, but yes, I'm back to fully leaded coffee, a couple of pots per day."

"Well, at least you don't smoke or dip tobacco," said the doctor, "but between your caffeine and alcohol, I'm not surprised you're still having reflux symptoms. It sounds like alcohol is the most likely cause for your abnormal liver tests. Since there is nothing else abnormal in your physical exam or the rest of your bloodwork, let's have you abstain from alcohol for about ten days, and then we'll repeat your lab. Enjoy the fall colors," she added, handing Luke his lab slip, "and I'll see you back late next week."

The ten days passed quickly for Luke. During the days, he enjoyed exploring new hikes with Stash, watching the dog scout for deer and small mammals as he followed his keen nose off the trails. Late afternoons and evenings were tied up with work on the computer, slugging down mugs of special blends from his favorite local coffee shop, Camp 4 Coffee. Although he found it a bit difficult to wind down at the end of the night without his evening drink, the natural discipline that had carried him to corporate success kicked in, and Luke strictly followed the doctor's advice. "See you next week," he said, patting the door to the wine cellar on his way past.

Back in the doctor's office, Luke and Dr. Joanne were both disappointed by his blood test results. "Your liver functions are still significantly elevated, Luke, so now we need to start looking for other causes," said the doctor.

"You sound so serious. How bad can it be, with everything else being normal?" asked Luke.

Dr. Joanne was very pragmatic. "First, we'll send out your blood to test for the different types of infectious hepatitis. I know you've had the hepatitis B series of shots, but we'll make sure your antibodies show immunity, plus we'll check for hepatitis C and A. Type A is unlikely, since your enzymes have been abnormal for a couple years, and type A doesn't go on to cause long term problems."

"Were the hepatitis B shots the ones I got before traveling to China a few years ago?"

"Yes, by my notes in your chart, it looks like you received those in California around four years ago."

"Are those vaccines very effective?" he asked.

"Absolutely. Hepatitis B is an enormous global health problem. More than two billion people worldwide have been infected, and of that group, more than three hundred and fifty million people have become chronic carriers of the infection. Complications of the infection account for over a million deaths annually. The hepatitis B vaccine is ninety-five percent effective in preventing chronic infections from developing. Here in the United States, there are more than a million carriers of hepatitis B, but since we recommended universal vaccination of children in 1991, the overall rate of acute cases of hepatitis B has dropped nearly seventy percent, and almost ninety percent in children and adolescents."

"That's impressive. So hopefully, for me this means that I shouldn't have hepatitis B. Is there anything else you need to test?" asked Luke.

"We'll also check for HIV, although according to your history you are low risk, with no drug use, no prior STDs, and only a few prior sexual partners," Dr. Joanne said, referring to notes in the chart. "Unless there's been any change in that lately?" she asked.

"Hardly," Luke replied. "Truthfully, relationships take too much time. I've always been kind of an introvert, and in general, I'm happier by myself or hanging out with my Stash."

"Referring to your dog, not drugs, right?" Dr. Joanne laughed, "Because that would definitely change your risk factors."

"Absolutely," confirmed Luke.

"Anyway, since you have a completely normal white blood cell count and no physical complaints, it's unlikely to be a mono syndrome, which is something else that can cause transient liver function abnormalities."

"Are there any other tests besides bloodwork?" he asked.

"If these tests all come back normal, then we'll have you get an abdominal ultrasound."

"What's that for?" asked Luke.

"It would provide a good look at your liver and your gallbladder. Sometimes, gallstone disease will cause liver function abnormalities, even without symptoms. Let's take it one step at a time though, Luke. We'll get your extra blood tests back in a few days, and we'll go from there, okay?"

"All right," agreed Luke. "You know, maybe it's my caffeine. I'll switch to decaf and see if that makes any difference while we're waiting on the other results."

"It certainly won't hurt, Luke, except possibly for the withdrawal headache," she smiled wryly.

The next Monday, Luke was back in the exam room again. Dr. Joanne came in and sat down with a concerned look on her face.

"Luke, it looks like we've got an answer to why your liver enzymes are abnormal. Your hepatitis C antibody test came back positive."

"Meaning that I've got hepatitis C?" echoed Luke skeptically.

"Yes, I'm afraid so."

"Seriously? I thought only drug addicts got that," exclaimed Luke.

"Well, people who use IV drugs certainly are at high risk for it, but up to twenty percent of people with hepatitis C have no identifiable risk factor except intercourse."

"Sex, huh?" retorted Luke.

Dr. Joanne continued, "On the plus side, your tests showed that your body has immunity to types A and B, so we don't need to worry about getting you up to speed on those shots," she commented.

"Why does that matter?" asked Luke.

"If a person develops one type of hepatitis, we immunize them against the other types to minimize any potential further damage to the liver," explained Dr. Joanne.

"Makes sense," Luke agreed.

Dr. Joanne looked back at the lab results. "Another bit of good news is that your HIV test was negative."

"I'd hope so," Luke remarked flippantly. "So, cut to the chase. What does this mean? Can you treat me?"

Dr. Joanne shook her head. "No. I'm going to refer you to a gastrointestinal specialist in Colorado Springs. Dr. Swegler specializes in liver diseases, especially hepatitis C. You may not even need any treatment now, but I'd like you to get established with someone in Colorado if you're going to be up here more permanently. Either that or you can see someone back in California. We're too small locally to have this kind of specialist here."

"What will he do for me?" asked Luke.

"*She* will do some additional tests to decide if you meet the criteria for treatment, possibly including a liver biopsy," replied Dr. Joanne.

"That doesn't sound too fun," commented Luke. "Can't you tell how bad the disease is by my liver enzymes?"

"No, the enzyme levels actually do not correlate well with how severe the hepatitis C infection is," said the doctor.

"Even though they went back to normal for awhile, before they went up again? It seems to me that should be a good sign," rationalized Luke.

"That would sound logical, but with hepatitis C, the blood enzyme levels can fluctuate up and down irregardless of the disease progression."

"Is this a really bad disease? What's it going to do to me?"

"Well, like any chronic disease, there is a whole spectrum of how hepatitis C can appear," explained Dr. Joanne. She went on to say that more than three million Americans have chronic hepatitis C, with roughly thirty thousand new cases identified each year. Up to 80 percent of these people have no symptoms at all. Surprisingly, 15 to 30 percent of people infected with hepatitis C will spontaneously clear the virus and any liver damage within six months, for reasons unknown at this time. The other 70 to 85 percent will have persistent infection. If symptoms are present, they are usually vague, manifesting as fatigue, decreased appetite, muscle or joint aches, or abdominal discomfort.

"I assume you'll want to know the end point, Luke, so let me tell you that, typically, the disease takes up to twenty or thirty years to cause serious liver damage, with scarring called cirrhosis occurring in ten to twenty percent of chronic carriers. Drinking alcohol is the number one aggravating factor that accelerates this disease. Only one in twenty people who become chronic carriers will develop liver cancer, but liver cancer has a very high mortality rate. As a result, hepatitis C is the leading reason for liver transplantation in the United States."

Luke processed what Dr. Joanne had explained, then in his typical get-to-work attitude asked, "So what do we need to do now? Is there anything urgent? "

"Really, I'd simply advise you to avoid anything that is tough on the liver, so no products that contain acetaminophen, like Tylenol, and I'd recommend no alcohol."

"None, or moderation?" asked Luke hopefully.

"None. You've already got this hepatitis virus insulting your liver, so you want to avoid anything that will potentially further irritate it. When all's said and done, you basically want to do everything you can to maximize good health. That includes exercise, diet, and a positive attitude."

"Well, I'm positive I'll miss my wine," quipped Luke. "What else do I need to know about this? Is the only way to get this through sex?"

"Hepatitis C is transmitted by blood or body fluids. I know you don't do IV drugs, and you haven't had a blood transfusion, so presumably you caught this through sex. You can also get it by sharing razors or toothbrushes with someone who is infected, but it's still more likely from intercourse. Also, it's possible to get hepatitis C from tattoos, but unless I missed it, you don't have one, do you?" asked the doctor.

"No way, I can't stand needles," shuddered Luke.

"Obviously, you should let any prior partners know, so they can get tested, too," said Dr. Joanne.

"That'll be a great email, won't it?" said Luke sarcastically, "Hi, there. We haven't spoken in nearly ten years, but I simply wanted to say thanks for the disease you gave me."

"And any future partners," Dr. Joanne continued, choosing to ignore his remark. "Also, you shouldn't donate blood, semen, or organs."

"Again, the needle phobia," reminded Luke. "I never have donated blood, though I've always felt guilty about that, and I'd hope I'm not headed for organ donation any time soon."

"I'm just trying to be thorough," chastised Dr. Joanne. "You never know when a cousin might need a kidney or something."

"As long as you didn't mean organ donation after my imminent death," responded Luke.

"Absolutely not. Seriously, Luke, people with hepatitis C can remain asymptomatic for decades, and our treatments are getting better all the time. With your needle phobia, though, I do think I ought to tell you that one of the antiviral treatments, interferon, is actually in shot form."

"Great," remarked Luke sarcastically. "And what about that liver biopsy that you mentioned earlier? I'm assuming that involves a big needle," Luke tried to joke.

"That one is long, but skinny," smiled the doctor. "Seriously, though, let's not get ahead of ourselves. You may not even need a liver biopsy at this point. There is some controversy over the timing of liver biopsies in patients with hepatitis C. Your liver enzymes are moderately elevated, but you have no other bloodwork abnormalities, and you don't have any physical findings that suggest advancing liver disease. It will be up to your liver specialist to determine whether or not they would recommend a liver biopsy at this point. I will tell you it is very individualized treatment, depending on both patient and doctor preference."

"So the doctor in Colorado might have a different opinion than one back in California?" asked Luke.

"Exactly. If I were you, I'd choose a gastrointestinal specialist in the state where you plan to spend the majority of your time for the next several years," suggested Dr. Joanne.

"For right now, I'd have to choose California, I guess," answered Luke. "Partly because I don't want to waste any time I've got up here trekking several hours over to Colorado Springs, but mainly because I need to be back in San Jose for probably six or seven months out of the next twelve."

"Let me know if you change your mind, and our office will get you Dr. Swegler's information over in the Springs," offered the doctor. "Do you have any other questions?"

"I hate to ask, but this whole thing came about because my new life insurance carrier found those high liver enzymes. They said that I would need clearance from my regular physician. I suppose we have to tell them that I've been diagnosed with hepatitis C, right?" asked Luke begrudgingly.

"Ethically, yes, that is the correct answer. You might want to wait until you see the liver specialist, so he or she can better assess your prognosis. I'd imagine that a life insurance company would not be too thrilled about this diagnosis, the same as they are not happy about any chronic disease. Every company is different, so I can't tell you how they will react specifically. I would assume this diagnosis may be grounds either to deny you coverage or to simply raise your rates," said Dr. Joanne.

"I'll be looking into it. Can I get a copy of all my labs from this month to take with me back to California?"

"Yes, I'll have the folks in the front get you a full set. Best of luck, Luke," wished Dr. Joanne, standing up and shaking his hand.

"Thanks, it sounds like I'll need it," responded Luke.

Back at home, Luke sat down in front of his computer, much to the disappointment of Stash, who was pawing at Luke's leg for attention and hoping for a walk. Luke rubbed Stash's head halfheartedly but focused his attention on his email address book. "I wonder if this email is even current," he mused as he clicked on the address of his old girlfriend. "She'll be surprised to hear from me outside of a Christmas card," Luke thought to himself.

Brenda was Luke's last serious girlfriend, and she seemed to harbor no ill will toward Luke, staying in touch with him through an annual exchange of Christmas cards. While Luke typically sent cards with offbeat holiday humor, Brenda's cards were classic family portraits, frequently involving Santa hats. She had become a university professor in biochemistry and was happily married to another Ph.D. Luke hoped she did not have this same veiled diagnosis. He typed "old friend" into the subject box and tabbed down to construct the email.

"Dear Brenda," he began. "What do I say?" thought Luke, rarely at a loss for words. His blunt, less-than-polished conversational style had never been his greatest asset. Luckily for him, his computer engineering skills and creative mathematical mind were the primary necessary tools for success in his world.

Luke moved the mouse and clicked back on the subject box, deleting "old friend" and entering "hepatitis C." He jumped back down to the text and kept it brief. "I'm feeling completely normal but have just been diagnosed with hepatitis C during some bloodwork for an insurance physical. My doctor suggested that I let any previous sexual partners know, so they can get screened too. No clue where I got this or how long I've had it. I hope it wasn't from you. Let me know, Luke."

Luke reread his note, and though the last couple lines didn't quite sound right, he clicked "send" before editing anything. The other two girls that he had slept with would be more challenging to locate.

Skye Smith was a girl that Luke had an off-and-on relationship with over several years. The last Luke had heard through the grapevine a few years back, Skye was doing some kind of volunteer work in Africa. Between her common last name and her global travels, Luke was doubtful of reaching her. He did a few web searches but only discovered links that were no longer current. That one would have to wait.

Finally, there was Ellen, the accountant. From his understanding of the timing of hepatitis C, it seemed more likely that he might have exposed Ellen than vice versa. Luke considered calling her but, frankly, didn't want the hassle. He settled instead for another succinct email. Under subject, he again listed "hepatitis C." Scrolling down, he typed, "Ellen, recent bloodwork showed I have hepatitis C. Doctors recommend that all my previous partners be tested."

But how should he sign it? "Sorry"? "Good luck"? "Sincerely"? Truly, nothing seemed appropriate. Luke remembered how Ellen used to say that she loved the diversion from her world of finance when her computer announced, "You've got mail."

"This email certainly won't bring a smile to her face. How will she react when she sees it?" Luke wondered. "At least I had it broken to me in stages," he reflected. However, Luke's pragmatic mindset kicked in at that point: "Well, it's the information that's important, not the acknowledgment." He merely added his name without any closing salutation. "After seeing the word 'hepatitis,' Ellen won't care about the rest, no matter what I say," Luke concluded, and with that thought, he clicked "send."

He leaned back, pushing away from his computer and stretching his arms. Stash jumped up, interpreting Luke's movements as a sign that it was time to head outside. He wagged his tail and looked up expectantly. Luke had originally intended to start work on some business proposals after he dashed off his personal emails, but distracted by Stash's reaction, he changed his plan.

"This hepatitis C mess is a lot to process, Stash. I think you've got the right idea. There's no point in trying to work right now." Luke stood up and grabbed the dog's leash. "Come on, let's go for a hike. The fresh air will do us both some good. I am not going to let this diagnosis rule my life," he affirmed. "Dr. Joanne said that I need to maximize my health, and I can't think of a better place to accomplish that than right here in these beautiful mountains. One challenge at a time, we'll conquer this. Let's go."

facts

Hepatitis C (HCV) Fact Sheet

What is it?

- Hepatitis C is an RNA virus, part of the hepatitis family, which includes hepatitis types A, B, C, D, and E.

How common is it?

- 3.2 million Americans (1.3% of the population) and 170 million people worldwide are infected with HCV.

How do you get it?

- Infected blood or body fluids transmit infection through transfusions, shared needles, or sexual intercourse, or from mother to fetus.

- Since 1992, screening for HCV has caused transfusion-related cases of HCV to drop to less than 1 per million units of blood.

- Sexual transmission of hepatitis C is thought to be inefficient, but. the actual percentage of any type of sexual transmission for hepatitis C is unknown. Up to 20% of people with hepatitis C have no known risk factor beyond intercourse.

Where on your body do you get it?

- HCV primarily infects the liver.

How do I know if I have it?

- 60 to 70% of people infected with HCV are asymptomatic.

- Blood tests check for antibodies to hepatitis A, B, and C.

- Hepatitis C is often a slowly progressive disease, lasting 10 to 40 years until serious liver damage occurs.

- One in ten people with HCV have no identifiable risk factors.

What does it look like?

- Usually there are no obvious visible signs of HCV infection.

- Jaundice—yellow eyes and skin—occurs in 20 to 30% of people with HCV.

What does it feel like?

- Many people feel completely normal.

- Nonspecific complaints of fatigue, nausea, loss of appetite, or abdominal pain occur in 10 to 20% of people with HCV.

- Headache, muscle aches, stiff neck, sore throat, fever, and flu-like symptoms can occur.

How long does it last?

- The incubation period, the time from exposure until the virus is detectable by laboratory testing, is 2 to 26 weeks.

- 70 to 85% of infections become chronic.

- Of chronic infections, 20% lead to cirrhosis (scarring of the liver).

- Of those with cirrhosis, 25% progress to liver failure.

- Once cirrhosis develops, the risk of getting hepatocellular (liver) cancer is 1 to 4% per year.

- Roughly 10,000 people die per year in the United States from complications of HCV.

Can it be cured?

- Not yet, although lasting clearance (meaning no detectable virus) can occur in 10 to 40% of infected patients treated with interferon and ribavirin. Relapse is not uncommon.

- Re-infection in transplanted livers is common.

What is the treatment?

- Current therapies involve three types of interferon, and combinations of interferon with ribavirin.

- These treatments can be associated with serious side effects, including depression, flu-like symptoms, nausea, headaches, and blood abnormalities.

How about alternative therapies?

- Stress reduction, healthy diet, and abstaining from alcohol help to improve overall health in patients with chronic hepatitis.

Are there long-term consequences?

- End-stage liver disease from HCV is the cause for over half of the liver transplants performed in the United States each year.

- 80% of HCV infections become chronic.

When are you contagious?

- Always.

Can hepatitis C be transmitted between homosexual partners?

- Yes. Exact transmission rates between homosexual partners, however, are unknown.

How do I avoid getting hepatitis C?

- Do not share needles.

- Do not share razors or toothbrushes.

- Do not use shared body-piercing equipment or tattoo needles.

- Abstain from sexual intercourse with partners with unknown hepatitis C status.

If I have hepatitis C, how do I avoid giving it to my partner?

- Do not share needles, razors, toothbrushes, or body-piercing equipment.

• Condoms decrease transmission of hepatitis C.

Frequently Asked Questions

➤ **Does one hepatitis vaccine prevent all types?**
No. The hepatitis A vaccine prevents only type A, and the hepatitis B vaccine only prevents type B. There is no vaccine for type C.

➤ **Can you get hepatitis C from kissing?**
No. HCV is not spread from kissing or casual contact.

➤ **Can you catch HCV from sharing razors?**
Yes. Razors, IV needles, acupuncture needles, tattoo needles, toothbrushes, or body-piercing equipment that have been used on a person with HCV can transmit the virus to another person.

➤ **If you are in a monogamous relationship with someone who has HCV, what is the chance you will catch it?**
Less than 1% per year, and less than 3% long-term, assuming you have no other risk factors.

Other co-existing STDs, particularly HIV disease, increase the risk of transmission significantly.

Higher risk sexual practices such as intercourse during menses or sexual activity that produces mucosal trauma can also increase transmission.

➤ **If a healthcare worker is stuck with a needle exposed to HCV, what is their chance of developing HCV infection?**
Approximately 2%.

Additional Information

American Liver Foundation
75 Maiden Lane, Suite 603
New York, NY 10038
1-800-GO LIVER (1-800-465-4837), or 201-256-2550
www.liverfoundation.org/

CDC-INFO
Centers for Disease Control and Prevention
1600 Clifton Road
Atlanta, GA 30333
1-800-CDC-INFO (1-800-232-4636), 1-888-232-6348 TTY
www.cdc.gov/ncidod/diseases/hepatitis/c/

HCV Advocate
Hepatitis C Support Project
P. O. Box 427037
San Francisco, CA 94142
www.hcvadvocate.org/

Hepatitis Foundation International
504 Blick Drive
Silver Spring, MD 20904
800-891-0707, or 201-239-1035
www.hepfi.org/

MedlinePlus
National Library of Medicine
8600 Rockville Pike
Bethesda, MD 20894
1-888-FIND-NLM (1-888-346-3656), or 301-594-5983
www.nlm.nih.gov/medlineplus/hepatitisc.html

SYPHILIS

18: Randy

RANDY SEARCHED THROUGH the magazines in the doctor's office lobby, pleasantly surprised to see a current issue of *Outdoor Life*. "Where is it?" he wondered, flipping quickly past the articles and lingering briefly over the advertisements. "Ah, yes, there I am," he smiled smugly to himself. "Look at those abs. Nice six-pack, if I do say so myself. Arms could use a little work, though," he thought critically. As Randy compared his biceps to the photo, he was dismayed once again at the red bumps covering his forearms and palms. "I sure hope we get an answer this time," he thought.

Randy depended on his physical appearance for his paycheck. Though he had been a model for years, Randy was trying to break into the acting business. His agent was fairly confident that Randy would get a second callback from his latest audition but had warned Randy that his rash had better be gone by then, or he would lose the part.

About two weeks ago, Randy began to notice small red circles on his palms after using a new moisturizing body lotion. The circles became bumps and quickly spread up his forearms. Randy had gone to a clinic, where he was given a steroid cream and told to stop using the new body lotion. Unfortunately, the rash not only didn't improve, it seemed to worsen in the next week. When Randy called back to the clinic for further advice, they referred him here to Dr. Kristyn, a dermatologist.

Randy had been slightly offended by her initially. Unlike his encounter at the previous clinic, Dr. Kristyn had put on gloves before examining his rash and had proceeded to ask him rather embarrassing questions.

"Randy, have you ever had any sexually transmitted diseases, and if so, which ones?" Dr. Kristyn had inquired.

"Well, yes," Randy had answered, though he didn't see the relevance to red bumps on his arms. "I've been treated for gonorrhea and chlamydia a couple times over the years, but never herpes," he added defensively.

"What about HIV or syphilis?" she had asked.

"No. I was last tested for HIV around a year ago, and it was negative," he replied proudly.

Dr. Kristyn took a small biopsy from his wrist area, assuring Randy that the scar would be minimal. She also ordered his blood drawn and asked Randy to follow up for the results in three days.

So here he sat, absentmindedly rubbing his arms, as was his recent habit, waiting to get some answers.

"Randy?" called the attractive blond medical assistant from the doorway.

Randy recognized her from his previous visit. "That's me, and you're Lorie, right?" Randy responded, flashing a winning smile in her direction and casually setting the magazine on the end table, still folded open to his ad.

Lorie coolly directed Randy into an exam room, not responding to his usually successful flirtatious banter. He pressed on, regardless. "Is that my results you've got clipped to the front of the chart? Come on, tell me what exotic disease I've got."

"Yes, it's your results, but no, it's not my job to discuss them. Dr. Kristyn will be in momentarily," Lorie replied curtly.

"Maybe I'm losing my touch," Randy briefly mused. Lorie had seemed interested in him earlier in the week but was clearly giving him the cold shoulder today. "Nah, she must be having a bad day," he decided.

Dr. Kristyn entered shortly after Lorie left and cut right to the chase as she sat down in front of Randy. "Well, my suspicions were correct. Randy, you have syphilis, secondary syphilis, to be exact."

"On my hands?" Randy recoiled. "Don't you get that on your, uh, privates?"

"Yes, that is typically the location of the initial lesion," said the doctor.

"But I haven't had any red bumps down there, and believe me, I would know," said Randy defensively.

"Actually, you'd be surprised how often people don't know they have STDs," responded Dr. Kristyn. "In the case of syphilis, the initial lesion is usually a single, painless ulcer that shows up anywhere from nine to thirty days after exposure and lasts from three to six weeks. It's most often on the penis in men, but it could have been in your mouth, where you might not have noticed it. Have you had any new sexual partners in the last few months?"

"Plenty, but no one gets syphilis anymore," protested Randy.

"I'll grant you that it's the least common sexually transmitted disease in the United States, but there are still around eight thousand cases per year reported," said Dr. Kristyn.

"So I got lucky?" Randy tried to joke.

"Frankly, yes. Most of the cases of syphilis that we see now are found in patients who have HIV disease, but your HIV test came back negative. Syphilis we can cure, HIV we cannot," responded Dr. Kristyn matter-of-factly.

"Thank goodness for small favors," Randy smirked. "So what's the cure?"

"Plain, old-fashioned penicillin," answered Dr. Kristyn.

"So what about this rash? I still don't get how a rash on my arms is from syphilis," doubted Randy.

"Well, the first lesion of syphilis is that painless ulcer, but even if it is untreated, that initial spot will heal. If proper antibiotics are not taken, syphilis then emerges as what you've got, secondary syphilis, which is typically non-itchy red marks and bumps on the skin, especially on the palms or soles. That was the clue for me to check for syphilis, by the way. Not too many rashes involve the palms. The timing with your lotion threw off your first examiner, but I had the benefit of seeing that steroids didn't help and was able to think a little broader," she said modestly.

"And what would have happened if I didn't come in now?" Randy pursued.

"Actually, the rash would have eventually disappeared, but it often recurs," explained the doctor. "The worst part is that you can develop tertiary syphilis, which can enter your brain and other organs, causing mental illness, deafness, blindness, and/or death. They call syphilis the great imitator, because when it gets to that stage, it can look like many other diseases."

"Then I guess I am lucky that I came in," said Randy. "So you're telling me that penicillin will make my rash go away and never come back, and I won't develop any of these worse signs of syphilis?"

"That's correct, with one caveat," Dr. Kristyn answered.

"And what's that?"

"That you don't get re-infected," replied the doctor. "Having syphilis once does not protect you from getting it again. It sounds like you're unsure where you caught it, so if you have unprotected sex of any type, you can catch it again. Please advise any sexual partners you've had within the last several months that they must get tested and treated to stop the spread of this disease. Also, since you have secondary syphilis, you need to know that those red bumps are teeming with the bacteria that cause syphilis, so there is the potential to have infected people who have touched them."

"Including the people at the first clinic?" Randy asked with surprise.

"In theory, anyone who touched your rash without wearing gloves, especially if they had any breaks in their skin," confirmed Dr. Kristyn.

"Actually, they may be the only ones," mused Randy. "I've been so self-conscious about this rash that I've been covering it up most of the time."

"I'd suggest you go back to your regular doctor anyway, to be tested for all of the sexually transmitted diseases as well as for follow-up blood tests for both HIV and syphilis. I'd also suggest you refrain from unprotected intimacy in the future." Dr. Kristyn finished, "Lorie will be back in with your penicillin shot and a handout on syphilis and other STDs."

Randy chuckled at the thought of Lorie returning. "No wonder she was aloof today," he reasoned. "Really, though, what's the big deal? As they say, I've got nothing penicillin won't cure, and once this rash is gone, who wouldn't want a piece of this?" Randy arrogantly concluded.

Lorie, for her part, could no longer see the handsome stud she had flirted with earlier in the week. When she administered the penicillin shot, all Lorie could perceive was a conceited model who had clearly slept with at least one person too many.

19: Liz

"THANK YOU, EVERYONE, AND good night. Look for us next week at Club Heat!" Liz croaked into the microphone over the exuberant crowd. To herself, she added, "Yeah, Club Heat, where I'll be puking in between sets if this so-called morning sickness doesn't let up."

"Great jamming on that last song, Lizzy," congratulated Zane, her boyfriend and the lead guitarist in their band.

"Yeah, you should be pregnant more often," joked the drummer, Rex. "I think it makes your voice sexy, and everyone's definitely loving your new cleavage."

Liz rolled her eyes at Rex, retorting, "My voice is husky from throwing up, and before you know it, my belly will be bigger than my breasts, so enjoy it while you can. Pregnancy is not so great from my end."

"Hey, Liz, careful what you say. That's my little rock star you've got cooking in there," teased Zane.

"Well, our little rock star better start letting me get some rest," Liz answered. Glancing at her watch, she added, "Speaking of rest, are you coming with me to my doctor's appointment in six hours?"

Zane groaned. "What were you thinking, getting an eight o'clock appointment when we have a late gig the night before?"

"I'm thinking that's the time they asked me to come in when they called on Friday, and since they're squeezing me in, I can't be choosy," snapped Liz.

"Fine, I'll go. Do we get to see the little rocker this time?" Zane asked.

"I have no idea, but I'll bet we'll at least hear his heartbeat again," said Liz, packing away her guitar and handing the case to Zane. "Thanks for carrying my other baby."

"Anything for you, babe," Zane smiled.

Only a few hours later, Liz was sitting in the obstetrician's exam room waiting for the doctor. She had decided to let Zane sleep in, knowing he had to be at his day job at noon and really needed the rest. Liz was napping on the exam table when the doctor finally arrived.

"Sorry for the wait, I had an emergency delivery," Dr. Garcia apologized as she entered.

"No problem, I needed the rest," smiled Liz.

"Is the morning sickness easing up yet?" asked the doctor.

"Actually, it's minimal in the mornings, but afternoons and nights are pretty tough," admitted Liz.

"Well, hang in there. You're almost past the first trimester, so it should get better soon," said Dr. Garcia. "Now, we called you back in because there was a problem on your initial blood tests, Liz. Unfortunately, you apparently have syphilis."

Liz laughed, "Yeah, right."

"It's not a laughing matter, Liz, I'm serious," chastised the doctor.

Liz sat up straight, "Are you for real? How can I have syphilis and not know it?"

"Actually, it's pretty common for people to be unaware of syphilis. That's one reason it's a required test for all pregnant women. Luckily, the rest of your screening tests—HIV, hepatitis C, gonorrhea, and chlamydia—were all negative. The first sign of syphilis is a sore in the vagina, anus, or mouth, but it's painless and goes away on its own, so many people are unaware of it. Although the ulcer goes away, the infection persists, and the second stage of syphilis is a rash that can come and go for weeks, usually on the hands," explained Dr. Garcia.

"Oh, man, I had a rash on my palms all last spring," exclaimed Liz. "We thought it was from my new guitar, and Zane said he'd had the same kind of thing before, so I ignored it, since it didn't itch or hurt. Besides, it finally went away."

"And Zane is?"

"My boyfriend, the baby's father. So you think I got it from him? What's it going to do to the baby?" Liz asked anxiously. "He should have come, after all."

"Okay, one step at a time," Dr. Garcia said. "First of all, yes, it sounds like you may have contracted syphilis from him. To be sure, he needs to see his doctor to be tested and treated, and you both need to abstain from sex until you are both treated to be sure you don't get re-infected."

"Okay," agreed Liz.

"Secondly, it sounds like you have what we call latent syphilis, meaning that you have no signs or symptoms of syphilis but you still harbor the infection inside you, where it could go on to cause serious damage in the future if it were untreated. Fortunately, the cure for you is simple—a shot of penicillin today and possibly another penicillin shot later because you are pregnant. The hope is that the penicillin will also completely treat your baby," explained the obstetrician.

"And if it doesn't?" Liz asked fearfully.

"Well, untreated syphilis in pregnancy has up to a forty percent chance of causing miscarriage. Syphilis can also cause blood problems, premature births, or congenital syphilis in the newborn, meaning the baby can develop multiple problems including seizures, developmental delays, and problems with its liver, spleen, or nervous system," explained the doctor.

"But, as long as we treat this now . . ." began Liz.

"We're hopeful that the baby will be fine. We'll be following blood tests on you throughout your pregnancy to make sure that your treatment looks successful, and we'll be able to look closely at your baby with an ultrasound later in pregnancy to check on him or her," reassured Dr. Garcia.

"Can the penicillin hurt the baby at all?" asked Liz.

"Typically not at this stage of pregnancy. Rarely, the penicillin can trigger a reaction that can lead to miscarriage, but the risk of untreated syphilis is much greater," she explained.

Liz chewed on her lip while she absorbed the information. "So there's no guarantee that my baby will be healthy," she asserted.

Dr. Garcia placed her hand gently on Liz's arm, saying, "No, Liz, there's not, but there never is. Babies can have defects that no one can predict, but we do screening tests like the syphilis test to find and treat everything that we can. That's what prenatal care is all about. Now, unless you have any more questions, I'll send in my nurse with your shot. Please make sure that your boyfriend gets to a doctor and so do any other sexual partners you may have had during the last year or so. If you had the rash last spring, you likely contracted syphilis a couple of months before that."

"Got it," murmured Liz, tears forming and starting to spill down her cheeks.

"I know it sounds stupid," Liz added tremulously, "but it never occurred to me that there could be something wrong with the baby. I mean, we even didn't plan for this pregnancy, but we figured we could handle it. But now, if there're serious problems...Could I please hear the heartbeat before you leave?"

Dr. Garcia reached for the Doppler, and squeezing jelly on Liz's lower abdomen, quickly picked up the high-pitched, rhythmic whooshing of the baby's heart. "Welcome to parenting, Liz. It's never what you expect."

facts

Syphilis Fact Sheet

What is it?

- Syphilis is caused by a bacterium called *Treponema pallidum*.

How common is it?

- It is the least common sexually transmitted disease in the United States. During 2006, there were 9,756 reported cases of primary and secondary syphilis and 36,935 total cases (including primary, secondary, latent, and tertiary syphilis).

- The year 1990 had the peak number of total cases of syphilis in the United States over the last fifty years, at 135,590 cases.

- African Americans have the highest rates compared with Hispanics and Caucasians, at 11.3, 3.6, and 1.9 cases per 100,000 people in the CDC's 2006 statistics.

- Males contract syphilis at a rate 5.7 times greater than females.

- Syphilis is often linked with HIV disease.

How do you get it?

- Syphilis is transmitted through sexual contact—oral, anal, or vaginal—with an infected person.

- Syphilis can be passed from a mother to her unborn child, causing congenital syphilis.

Where on your body do you get it?

- There are four distinct stages of syphilis:
  - The first, or "primary" syphilis infection shows up as a small, firm, painless round ulcer, called a chancre, at the site where the bacterium entered the body. These ulcers are usually located on the penis, labia, or vagina, but can also occur on the cervix, in the anus, or in the mouth.
  - "Secondary" syphilis typically presents as a non-itchy skin rash, often present on the palms or soles of the feet but sometimes covering more of the body.
  - "Latent" syphilis is untreated syphilis without obvious symptoms.
  - "Tertiary" syphilis can show up anywhere in the body, causing a variety of symptoms including deafness, blindness, mental illness, heart disease, neurological disorders, and death.

How do I know if I have it?

- Many people are unaware of the initial ulcer because it is painless and can be in a location that can't be easily seen. The ulcer will go away with or without treatment, but the infection remains and may progress.

- If you have a genital ulcer, especially one followed by a rash, a medical professional should examine you and check for syphilis.

- Blood tests can reveal the presence of infection; the blood tests RPR, VDRL, and FTA all check for antibodies to syphilis.

- A swab of an ulcer can reveal syphilis when viewed under a dark field in the microscope.

What does it look like?

- Primary syphilis is usually a single small, firm, round ulcer on the vagina, labia, penis, or less often, the mouth or other body location.

- Secondary syphilis looks like red spots on the palms or soles.

- Tertiary syphilis is called the "great imitator" because it can look like such a variety of diseases, depending on which system it affects.

What does it feel like?

- The ulcers of syphilis are typically painless.

- The rash is often not itchy.

- In secondary syphilis, there can be nonspecific symptoms such as mild sore throat, fatigue, headache, and swollen lymph nodes.

How long does it last?

- Primary syphilis usually breaks out about 3 weeks after exposure but can range from 9 to 30 days after exposure.

- The chancre will last from 3 to 6 weeks and then will disappear with or without treatment. The infection will persist even when the ulcer leaves, unless antibiotics are used.

- The rash of secondary syphilis occurs 2 to 10 weeks after the chancre appears, often after the chancre is completely gone. The rash will disappear without treatment but often recurs. Again, the infection will persist unless antibiotics are given.

Can it be cured?

- Yes.

What is the treatment?

- Penicillin is still the treatment of choice for syphilis.

- For people allergic to penicillin, there are alternative antibiotics.

How about alternative therapies?

- No herbs or over-the-counter treatments are effective for syphilis.

Are there long-term consequences?

- Untreated syphilis can lead to neurosyphilis and other forms of tertiary syphilis.

- Tertiary syphilis can cause deafness, blindness, mental illness, heart disease, and death.

When are you contagious?

- Once infected, you are contagious until you are cured with antibiotics. Latent syphilis is the least contagious; primary, secondary, and early latent syphilis are the most contagious.

Can syphilis be transmitted between homosexual partners?

- According to 2006 CDC data, 64% of all new cases of primary and secondary syphilis in the United States occurred in homosexual men.

- There is a case report of woman-to-woman transmission, but this is not thought to be common.

How do I avoid getting syphilis?

- Abstinence from oral, anal, and vaginal intercourse will prevent transmission of primary syphilis.

- Condoms reduce (but do not eliminate) transmission of syphilis only when they cover an active sore. However, lesions are frequently outside the area sheathed by a condom.

- Secondary syphilis can be contracted through skin-to-skin contact with an infected person; be especially cautious of rashes on people's palms or soles.

If I have syphilis, how do I avoid giving it to my partner?

- Abstain from oral, anal, and vaginal intercourse until both you and your partner have been fully treated for syphilis with appropriate antibiotics.

Frequently Asked Questions

➤ Can you catch syphilis from a toilet seat?
No. The bacterium dies when it gets dry.

➤ Since syphilis has been around for centuries, is it resistant to most antibiotics?
No. Syphilis still responds to penicillin and other antibiotics.

➤ **Can you have syphilis and not know it?**
Yes, particularly since the initial sores are not painful and often not easily visible.

➤ **Have any famous people suffered from syphilis?**
King Henry VIII, Al Capone, Friedrich Nietzsche, and Franz Schubert, to name a few.

➤ **When are people tested for syphilis?**
Many states require a blood test for syphilis to obtain a marriage license, and pregnant women are tested to prevent congenital syphilis in their babies.

Additional Information

American Social Health Association
P. O. Box 13827
Research Triangle Park, NC 27709
1-800-783-9877
www.ashastd.org/learn/learn_syphilis.cfm

CDC-INFO
Centers for Disease Control and Prevention
1600 Clifton Road
Atlanta, GA 30333
1-800-CDC-INFO (1-800-232-4636), 1-888-232-6348 TTY
www.cdc.gov/std/syphilis/default.htm

MedlinePlus
National Library of Medicine
8600 Rockville Pike
Bethesda, MD 20894
1-888-FIND-NLM (1-888-346-3656), or 301-594-5983
www.nlm.nih.gov/medlineplus/syphilis.html

20 : Elaine's Epilogue

ELAINE WAS EXHAUSTED. It had been three nights since she had been able to get any decent sleep. On Tuesday night, she had been up tending to her younger daughter, Catherine, who had a stomach virus. Wednesday night, Elaine had been on call for her family practice group of six physicians, and with flu season in full gear, the beeper seemed to go off every fifteen minutes all night long. Last night, all she had wanted to do was get to bed early, but her husband, Matt, had been on call at the hospital for his cardiology group. This left Elaine parenting the kids by herself on a night filled with soccer practice, make-up homework, and a science-fair project. Elaine had finally made it to bed around eleven thirty, which left her only six hours to get caught up on sleep before Friday's routine began.

The morning schedule had been packed with the usual mix of patients: people with diabetes, high blood pressure, or depression, as well as everyone with a cough who wanted to be fixed for their weekend activities. Elaine looked at the remaining two patients on her schedule. The first was a teenager with a skin problem, and the second was a new patient with a sore throat. "Good," she thought.

They should both be quick. She glanced down at her watch and was dismayed that it was already two thirty. That would leave her less than forty-five minutes to see these last patients, finish writing all her charts from the day, and review lab results before she needed to leave to pick up her kids from school.

Elaine rarely drank caffeine, but she was craving a pick-me-up to help her through the last hour. She ducked into the break room and grabbed a soda from the fridge. Since the next patient wasn't ready yet, Elaine sat down and started writing her notes in the charts as she drank her soda. Suddenly, Elaine realized that she had been ignoring a growing tingling sensation on the right side of her crotch. "Oh, man, not today," she thought as her heart sank. But really, it was no surprise after the week she'd had. Elaine now had over a decade of personal experience dealing with genital herpes, so she had no doubt what it meant when she started feeling burning and tingling on that right side.

It seemed a lifetime ago that she had been a first-year medical student diagnosed with herpes. The first two years had been completely awful. Between lack of sleep, crummy nutrition, and tons of stress, Elaine constantly had outbreaks, even after she started taking daily preventative medicines. In fairness, with her call schedule, working thirty-six hour shifts and losing track of time and days, she had not been able to take the medicines as consistently as she should have. She had to be sure to wear loose cotton underwear, and she had avoided wearing jeans throughout the rest of med school. During her residency, the outbreaks had decreased to every three or four months.

Elaine had dated several different guys during medical school but chose not to be intimate with anyone again until she fell head over heels in love with Matt. She remembered her relief when she had the painful discussion with Matt about her disease and found out that he, too, had a history of genital herpes, which he got when he was in college. Luckily for him, he had only a couple of outbreaks the year he caught it and never had another problem with it. She and Matt had been married for twelve years.

Elaine thought about the C-sections she had to have when her children were born because of having an outbreak when she went into labor with her first child. This disease had impacted her life for a long time. She picked up her purse and fished through it until she found her prescription medications. She was happy that it had been almost a year since her last outbreak. Elaine still carried the pills in her purse from force of habit but had rarely needed them these past several years. She swallowed the pill along with the last of her soda just as her nurse, Vicki, walked around the corner.

"Your next patient is ready," Vicki announced. Then in a quieter voice, she added, "This one might take a bit longer than we originally thought."

Elaine stood up and took the chart from her nurse. "Isn't this the teenager with acne? Is it that bad?" she asked.

"Not acne. Her skin problem is on her bottom," said the nurse. "By the way, her mom is with her today."

Elaine exchanged a look of resignation with Vicki and headed down the hallway toward the patient.

"Hi, Meg. Hi, Mrs. Schmid. So, how have you been doing?" Elaine asked.

Meg was a volleyball star at a nearby high school. Elaine had taken care of her since her early grade-school years but had probably seen her only twice per year on average—once each year for her annual sports-participation physical and sometimes again for an injury or a minor illness. Elaine was trying to remember if Meg had mentioned having a boyfriend during her physical last summer.

"I'm doing great, except for this skin thing," replied Meg.

"Yes, she has what looks like a spider bite or something," her mom added. "I gave her some antibiotic cream to put on it earlier in the week, but it doesn't look any better to me. I think she's making it worse by scratching it."

"I'm not scratching it, Mom. It doesn't itch, it kind of stings," said Meg.

"All right. So Meg, when did you first notice it?" asked Elaine.

"I think it first started last weekend as a little red bump," said Meg.

"But when you showed me on Tuesday, it looked more like several bites," interjected her mom, "and now it's kind of crusted, like it's infected."

"Well, the last time I had one, it looked just like this, and it went away on its own," Meg replied defensively.

"You've had this before?" both Elaine and Mrs. Schmid said, almost at the same time.

"Yeah, I had a bite like this last semester, but it was higher up, so it didn't rub on my underwear as much. I guess that's why it wasn't as bad," said Meg.

"Have you had these bumps anywhere else on your body?"

"No, just on the right side of my booty," said Elaine.

"Okay. Well, with skin things, a picture is worth a thousand words, so let's take a look, okay?" asked Elaine.

"Sure," said Meg, reaching down to pull the gown away.

Elaine interrupted her. "Just a minute. Meg, would you like your mom to stay, or would you prefer more privacy?" Elaine turned and looked toward Mrs. Schmid. "No offense, of course. I just always like to offer that to teenagers." She was trying to keep her voice light but wanted to communicate with Meg that she might be bringing up issues that could be uncomfortable to discuss with her mom present. Meg's mom picked up what was going on immediately, although Meg clearly did not.

"Meg, would you like me to leave? Is there anything you need to discuss in private with the doctor?" she asked intently, leaning forward and looking her daughter straight in the eyes.

Meg shrugged her shoulders and with a quick roll of her eyes said, "Whatever, Mom. It's no big deal." Then she looked at Elaine. "Really, it's just a bug bite, or rash, or whatever."

Elaine pulled on a pair of gloves. She walked over to the exam table and asked Meg to go ahead and lie back. Elaine lifted the gown and looked down at Meg's bottom. Sure enough, she saw exactly what she was expecting—a cluster of scabbed-over blisters on a bright red base. She also saw a circular dark area higher up on the same side. "Is this where the last one was?" she asked.

Meg twisted her body so she could look where Elaine was pointing. "Yeah, right there where that dark spot is now."

Elaine tried to be casual. She swabbed the area with the cotton-tipped applicator from the herpes culture kit as she asked, "So, have you noticed any vaginal discharge or irritation with these?"

Meg blushed. "No."

"Okay, then, go ahead and sit up, and let's talk about this for a minute," said Elaine.

Before Elaine could say anything else, Mrs. Schmid jumped in. "Meg, have you and Daniel been sleeping together?" she asked in a level voice.

Now Meg was bright red but emphatic. "No. We absolutely have not had sex, Mom."

Elaine felt like disappearing. She had no doubt that this was herpes. The only question was how to handle the situation with Meg's mom present. Elaine preferred to deal with the underage patient one on one and then help that patient find a way to communicate the information to the parent.

Luckily, at this point, Meg's mom stood up, clearly struggling with mixed emotions, and very quietly and calmly said, "You know what? I think I would prefer it if the two of you discussed Meg's rash alone, and then I'll come back in and you can explain it to me in a few minutes, okay?"

Meg offered up a mild protest but looked relieved when her mom was gone.

After the door closed, Elaine looked at Meg.

"I swear, we have not had sex yet. What is the deal? What do you think this is?" she rattled off.

Elaine took a breath. "Well, it certainly looks like herpes." She paused a moment while Meg looked at her in shock, tears filling her eyes.

"But really, we have not had sex," she cried.

"Meg," Elaine said calmly, "have you had oral sex?"

Meg had now lost all composure. "Yes, just a few times, but that doesn't count, does it?" she sobbed.

"Unfortunately, it does count for this. If he had herpes in his mouth, which is really common, then you could have caught this from oral sex," Elaine explained.

"But, it's on my rear end, not my front. Trust me, he didn't go there," Meg insisted.

"The herpes virus comes in through the skin but then goes to the nervous system," explained Elaine. "When it comes out, it picks one nerve route to travel on, which is why it stays on one side. Most of the time, it does show up a little closer to the labia or vagina, but often it appears on either the front of the leg or on the rear end, where you have it."

Meg bit her lip and tried to process what she was hearing. Elaine knew only too well what was going on in her brain. Elaine partly wanted to hug her, tell Meg that she herself had gotten this disease the exact same way, and share how she had coped with it. Part of her wanted to maintain her professional distance, and truthfully, part of her just wanted to finish up so she could go get her kids and escape this painful part of her job. In the end, her natural compassion won out, and she told Meg the story of her "best friend Stephanie" in medical school who had suffered from herpes but had learned to deal with it. She taught Meg all about the disease and its treatment and prevention. Elaine talked to Meg at length about birth control and other sexually transmittable diseases, though Meg swore that after this, she would never be intimate with her boyfriend again. Finally, Elaine asked what Meg would like Elaine to tell her mother.

This brought more tears, but Meg composed herself fairly quickly and said with far more maturity than Elaine thought that she would have had at seventeen, "You know, I got myself into this. I should be the one to tell her. Will you stay here while I tell her, so you can answer any questions she has?"

"Of course," Elaine answered.

She stepped out of the room and asked the nurse to bring back Meg's mom. As Elaine checked her watch, Vicki said, "Don't worry, the last patient really is easy. I already did her rapid strep test, and it was positive. We'll get you out in time to get your kids if you take your charts with you."

"Thanks, Vicki, you're the best," said Elaine with a relieved smile.

She went back into the room, where Meg was already dressed and sitting on the end of the exam table. Mrs. Schmid entered just behind Elaine, and they both sat down. Meg didn't wait for any prompting. She looked right at her mom, and with tears still in her eyes, began pouring out her story. "Mom, I didn't lie. We haven't had sex, I promise. But we did get carried away and did, you know, have, um...oral sex a couple times last year. Please don't tell Dad, okay?" she ended in a rush.

Her mom looked as though she had been punched but, to her credit, remained calm. She looked at Elaine. "We'll have to talk about that later. Right now, let's just find out what we need to do for you." Mrs. Schmid turned her attention back to Elaine and asked, "So, what exactly is her rash?"

"It's herpes," Elaine replied.

"And can you give her an antibiotic to make it go away?" asked Mrs. Schmid.

Elaine went through most of her explanations about herpes again, concluding by handing Mrs. Schmid a prescription to be filled only if Meg had another breakout, since it was too late for the antiviral medicine to be helpful for this one. Elaine answered a few more questions and then gave them a handout to take home that contained all the information they had gone over. As Elaine walked out of the room, she was touched to see Mrs. Schmid get up and silently embrace her daughter in a tight hug. It always impressed her how many parents dealt well with bad news, at least in the office, despite what their children had expected.

As a parent herself, Elaine knew Mrs. Schmid had to be every bit as upset as Meg, although certainly with a different mix of emotions. Initial anger, fear, and disappointment would give way to the frustration of not being able to protect her daughter from this guy or this disease.

"What am I going to do to help protect my kids from ending up in a situation like this?" she thought. She hoped that raising the kids in a medical household would at least make it easier to talk about diseases when they were old enough to understand about sex. They actually understood many medical expressions like "respiratory distress" or "cardiac arrhythmias" from listening to their parents' conversations at home. Elaine chuckled as she pictured herself shifting the dinner conversation every night of their adolescence, telling story after story of unsuspecting young women and men catching these "gifts that keep on giving." Sadly, the real stories that her patients shared weekly had so many similarities that they seemed completely predictable to Elaine.

For example, what happens when a couple ends a long-term relationship, then sleeps together a month or two later for that "one last time" at a point when they are both just feeling lonely? Inevitably, one of them walks away from that reunion with a new disease. Or, when does a condom break? Exactly when the woman is ovulating, of course. Would it make a difference if her son and daughters really knew about these patterns and possibilities?

In Elaine's experience, it seemed that everyone believed only society's undesirables could have STDs. In reality, STDs have no bias. However wealthy, whatever race, however well educated a person may be, it doesn't matter. If you have sex, you're at risk for getting a sexually transmitted disease. "Just ask me," she thought, shaking her head as she walked down the hall to see her last patient. "Just ask me."

Bibliography

Bailey, J. V., C. Farquhar, C. Owen, and P. Mangtani. "STIs in Women Who Have Sex with Women." *Sexually Transmitted Infections* 80, no. 3 (2004).

Bauer, G. R., and S. Welles. "Beyond Assumptions of Negligible Risk: STDs and Women Who Have Sex with Women." *American Journal of Public Health.* 91, no. 8 (2001).

Beauman, John. "Genital Herpes: A Review." *American Family Physician* 72, no. 8 (2005).

Brown, D., and J. Frank. "Diagnosis and Management of Syphilis." *American Family Physician* 68, no. 2 (2003).

Campos-Outcalt, D., and S. Hurwitz. "Female-to-Female Transmission of Syphilis: A Case Report." *Sexually Transmitted Diseases* 29, no. 2 (2002).

Centers for Disease Control and Prevention. *HIV/AIDS Surveillance Report, 2006.* Vol. 18. Atlanta: U.S. Department of Health and Human Services, CDC, 2008. www.cdc.gov/hiv/topics/surveillance/resources/reports/.

————. "Sexually Transmitted Diseases Treatment Guidelines." *Morbidity and Mortality Weekly Report* 55 (2006).

————. "Updated Recommended Treatment Regimens for Gonococcal Infections and Associated Conditions—United States." *Morbidity and Mortality Weekly Report* 56 (2007).

Cram, L., M. Zapata, E. Toy, and B. Baker. "Genitourinary Infections and Their Association with Preterm Labor." *American Family Physician* 65, no. 2 (2002).

Fethers, K., C. Marks, A. Mindel, and C. Estcourt. "STIs and Risk Behaviours in Women Who Have Sex with Women." *Sexually Transmitted Infections* 76, no. 5 (2000).

Flinders, D., and P. De Schweinitz. "Pediculosis and Scabies." *American Family Physician* 69, no. 2 (2004).

Jin, F., et al. "Transmission of HSV Types 1 and 2 in a Prospective Cohort of HIV-negative Gay Men: The Health in Men Study." *Journal of Infectious Diseases* 194, no. 5 (2006): 561–70.

Khalsa, Ann. "Preventive Counseling, Screening, and Therapy for the Patient with Newly Diagnosed HIV Infection." *American Family Physician* 73, no. 2 (2006).

Kurowski, K. "The Woman with Dysuria." *American Family Physician* 57, no. 9 (1998).

Marr, Lisa. *Sexually Transmitted Diseases: A Physician Tells You What You Need to Know.* 2nd ed. Baltimore: Johns Hopkins University Press, 2007.

Marrazzo, J. M. "Genital HPV Infection in Women Who Have Sex with Women: A Concern for Patients and Providers. *AIDS Patient Care and STDs* 14, no. 8 (2000).

Marrazzo, J. M., K. Stine, and L. Koutsky. "Genital HPV Infection in Women Who Have Sex with Women: A Review." *American Journal of Obstetrics and Gynecology* 183, no. 3 (2000).

McMillan, A., and H. Young. "Rectal Chlamydial Infection among Men Who Have Sex with Men: Partner Notification as a Means of Nucleic Acid Amplification Test Validation." *International Journal of STD and AIDS* 18, no. 3 (2007).

Miller, K. "Diagnosis and Treatment of *Chlamydia trachomatis* Infection." *American Family Physician* 73, no. 8 (2006).

———. "Diagnosis and Treatment of *Neisseria gonorrhoeae* Infections." *American Family Physician* 73, no. 10 (2006).

Moran, J. "Clinical Evidence Concise—Gonorrhea." *American Family Physician* 72, no. 1 (2005).

Moyer, Linda, E. Mast, and M. Alter. "Hepatitis C: Part I. Routine Serologic Testing and Diagnosis." *American Family Physician* 59, no. 1 (1999).

———. "Hepatitis C: Part II. Prevention Counseling and Medical Evaluation." *American Family Physician* 59, no. 2 (1999).

Mravcak, S. "Primary Care for Lesbians and Bisexual Women." *American Family Physician* 74, no. 2 (2006).

Owen, M., and T. Clenney. "Management of Vaginitis." *American Family Physician* 70, no. 11 (2004).

Ribes, J., A. Steele, J. Seabolt, and D. Baker. "Six-Year Study of the Incidence of Herpes in Genital and Nongenital Cultures in a Central Kentucky Medical Center Patient Population." *Journal of Clinical Microbiology* 39, no. 9 (2001).

Roberts, C. M., J. R. Pfister, and S. J. Spear. "Increasing Proportion of Herpes Simplex Virus Type 1 as a Cause of Genital Herpes Infection in College Students." *Sexually Transmitted Diseases* 30, no. 10 (2003).

Shapley, M., J. Jordan, and P. Croft. "A Systematic Review of Postcoital Bleeding and Risk of Cervical Cancer." *British Journal of General Practice* 56 (June 2006): 453–60.

Smith, Liz. "ACOG Releases Guidelines for Managing Abnormal Cervical Cytology and Histology in Adolescents." *American Family Physician* 74, no. 8 (2006).

Temte, Jonathon. "HPV Vaccine: A Cornerstone of Female Health." *American Family Physician* 75, no. 1 (2007).

U.S. Preventive Services Task Force. "Screening for Chlamydial Infection: Recommendations and Rational." *American Family Physician* 65, no. 4 (2002).

Walsh, D. E., R. Griffith, and A. Behforooz. "Subjective Response to Lysine in the Therapy of Herpes Simplex." *Journal of Antimicrobial Chemotherapy* 12, no. 5 (1983).

Warner, L., et. al. "Condom Effectiveness for Reducing
    Transmission of Gonorrhea and Chlamydia: The Importance
    of Assessing Partner Infection Status." *American Journal of
    Epidemiology* 159, no. 3 (2004): 242–51.
Westrom, L., and P.-A. Mardh. "Acute Pelvic Inflammatory
    Disease (PID)." In *Sexually Transmitted Diseases,* 2nd ed., edited
    by K. K. Holmes, P.-A. Mardh, P. F. Sparling, and P. J. Wiesner,
    593–613. New York: McGraw-Hill, 1990.

Symptoms Index

Library of Congress Cataloging-in-Publication Data

Grimes, Jill.
   Seductive delusions : how everyday people catch STDs / Jill Grimes.
   p. cm.
   Includes bibliographical references and index.
   ISBN-13: 978-0-8018-9066-6 (hardcover : alk. paper)
   ISBN-13: 978-0-8018-9067-3 (pbk. : alk. paper)
   ISBN-10: 0-8018-9066-7 (hardcover : alk. paper)
   ISBN-10: 0-8018-9067-5 (pbk. : alk. paper)
   1. Sexually transmitted diseases—Popular works. 2. Self-care, Health. I. Title.
   RC200.G74 2008
   616.95'1—dc22   2008010645